LOVING THE FOODS I USE TO HATE!

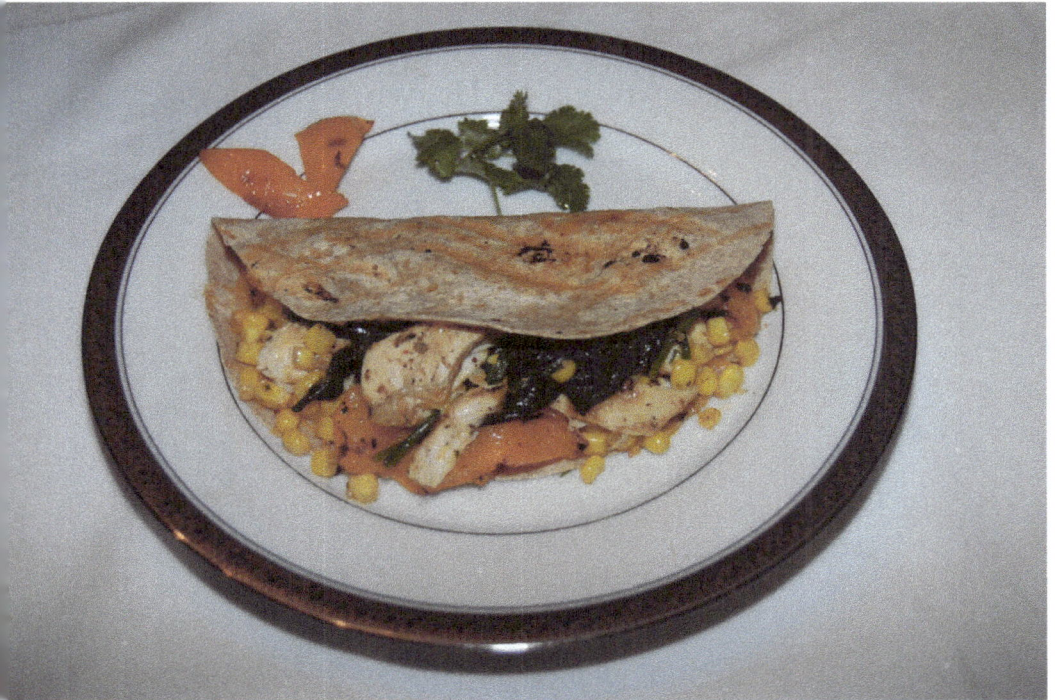

Living a Diabetic, Stress Free Life!

Author

Angela H. Brown

Publisher

Cherry Wine Publisher

Editor

Professhanel Editing

Table of Contents

Introduction

Have you ever felt like there is a sexy person just trapped inside of your body? If that applies to you, then I have developed a program that will change your life forever, because losing weight can be easy. Once I began my transformation, I began to look totally younger, and my life was renewed!

So many people approach me daily and ask, "What are you doing to lose all of that weight so quickly?" I never would have thought that someone would have asked me that question-EVER! Take a long look at your body and ask yourself, do I know what makes me gain or lose weight? I did. For years I was on a roller coaster ride; my body felt like a stranger.

Through the years I noticed that weight was coming on fast. I was three years in to my marriage, and my husband and I needed more room in our bed. We both got so comfortable with ourselves that food became the answer to all of our problems. In the eighth year of our marriage, my doctor told me that I was borderline diabetic, and he wanted me to lose the weight fast, before I became confined to medications or insulin shots. Needless to say, I was stunned and hurt, but the reality was that I needed to make some changes, and time was not on my side.

I waited a few months before I started on my journey, and I looked at myself in the mirror and *hated* what I saw. I no longer looked like myself; I was full of fluid, and my stomach was the size of a seven month pregnant woman! The next day I prayed to God to help me find what foods were best for me, and what foods would help me to lose the weight. I woke up with a new perspective on life, so I put on my boxing gloves and began to fight for my health! I decided, with the help of the

Lord, that if I didn't like what I saw, then I had to make the necessary changes.

This is an easy read; you only have to commit and stay focused. This book will lift your spirits and give you a new hope. Yes, there are so many books out there, but my book will help you learn how stress plays an important role in your weight. Take the stress test and learn how to fight those late night cravings. Losing the weight means losing the procrastination attitude, focusing on your goals, and having a winner attitude.

Some people settle for Mr. or Mrs. Wrong because they feel too insecure to have the man or woman of their dreams. No matter what size you are, you should be 100% healthy and ready to conquer the world. I will teach you how to love the foods that you hate and how great smells in the kitchen are *very* vital. You will also learn how to eat and how to live - not live to eat. Enjoy your new power house body and spread the word about good eating habits. Forget about dieting and imagine yourself on a new life style change!

Chapter 1
An Interview with Dr. Howard Nelson

In 2005 it was the best year of my life! I was planning a wedding with my very best friend, Mr. Perry C. Brown. At that time I was between a size eight and ten. My clothes fit just right and my health was in perfect condition. Perry asked me to be his wife and I accepted the offer, but no one told us that we would gain over 50 pounds each in the next five years. I have no regrets about the marriage, but Lord please take all of the unwanted pounds away!

The foods that I was eating were just sinful: pizza, seasoned wings, potato chips, baked chocolate chip cookies-yum yum and then some. After two years of our marriage, I noticed that my clothes were getting a little snug. Of course I ignored it; that was my job - to ignore the visible things. My husband and I hardly went anywhere except to visit family and to wine and dine one another. Food became our top choice for entertainment.

A few years into our marriage, I was beginning to notice that I needed new clothes. I was wearing tens and twelve's, and my mid-section was protruding past my upper thigh. Little by little I had started to become more tired and over worked. With all my business ideas and not having any investors, I became overwhelmed, which turned into stress. I had created this debt and there was no way out! So what was I to do?

We ate and binged, and the more we ate, the more miserable we became. Life became intense and food was my only comfort. The truth hurts and so do the unwanted pounds that people can carry around. My husband and I prayed and worried all the time. The good word says: if you pray then don't worry, and if you worry then don't pray (Matthew 6:25). Clearly we were not listening at all!

Couples can often begin to gain weight if the communication is not working in their relationship. My husband and I try to stay in prayer; because that is the only way we survive. Life itself can stress you out if you choose to not listen to your inner voice.

Life has its way of making you lose track of time. I recognized that the weight was coming on just by the bite of pizza. I soon became a size 14, borderline diabetic, and I sometimes had anxiety attacks; I became stagnant. As you begin to get older, you try to accept the fact that unusual things will happen to you. A client and dear friend of mine smiled and told me, "You know when you turn 40 everything will fall apart." That frightened me! I had no idea of how to beat those odds. I looked in to my own family and I thought: she just might be right! The road I was going down would make just certain that it would happen to me. One thing about my personality is that when someone tells me what I can't do, or if something negative might happen to me, I rebuke it!

I must admit, it took years before I got my wake up call. I remember the day I had a doctor's visit, and the nursing assistant weighted me. The scale all at once became a nightmare. I weighed a whopping 187 pounds; my heart *dropped*! Once I went into the doctor's office, he began consulting me, and all I could hear was a whisper of his voice. I was concentrating on what the nursing assistant had just told me - 187 pounds. I was only five-feet-two-inches tall! I was thinking, how did I get here, and Lord deliver me out of this fat suit. No way was I just going to accept this, but what was I going to do?

One night I remember staring in the mirror and my husband was looking me over like, boy I love her, but I know he was also thinking my baby has really gained some weight. I then began to slowly analyze my body. I looked seven months pregnant, but there was definitely not a baby in the oven. My husband looked helpless, but concerned; he knew that I was unhappy. That night I prayed and asked God to help me lose weight, and understand what makes my body lose and gain weight. I looked at myself that way for the last time. I had awakened and I was ready for a life change!

EXERCISE: YOUR WAKE UP CALL - THE STRESS TEST

Try this test to see if you're stressed out. If you answer yes to more than four of these questions, then you are stressed out. This is why many of us gain or lose too much weight.

1. Do you eat high fatty foods when you have problems?
2. Do you find your self crying or getting angered easily?
3. Do you have high-blood pressure?
4. Have you lost your job, or are you unable to travel due to financial stress?
5. Have you been divorced or having relationship problems?
6. Do you eat late at night and sleep on a full stomach?
7. Do you often experience stomach problems after you eat?
8. Do you find yourself thinking about food more than normal?
9. Have you gained over twenty pounds in the past five years?
10. When eating your meals, do you eat a lot of seconds and third helpings?
11. When entertaining with friends, do you often eat even if you're not hungry?
12. Do you drink alcohol weekly, taking in three or more drinks?
13. Do your children stress you out regularly?
14. Does your boss or coworkers stress you out?
15. Do you heavily season your food with high sodium?
16. Do you eat when you are bored?

Are you surprised at how stressed you are? Well don't feel bad, you can make a lifestyle change today!

Interview with Dr. Howard Nelson

I had the pleasure of sitting down with Dr. Howard Nelson, a 20 year Mental Health Practitioner in Memphis, Tennessee. Dr. Nelson has worked in a variety of positions including: providing alcohol and drug counseling, marital and family therapy, as well as individual therapy for children, adolescents and adults. Dr. Nelson shared with me the stress related issues that result in weight gain, and how stress actually plays a very important role in your hormones, as well as your weight. I really needed Dr. Nelson to clarify what makes the body gain and lose weight.

Q: Dr. Nelson, does stress play an important role in weight gain or weight lose?
A: Yes, Angela, there are two particular stresses: eustress, which is positive, and distress, which is negative. These stresses can be caused by getting married, losing a loved one, or getting a divorce. Anything that will cause you to over eat or not eat at all can be very stressful!

Q: Dr. Nelson, do you think there are people who are bipolar and may not know it?
A: Yes, many people are stressed out; some people have not been tested or diagnosed.

Q: Dr. Nelson, how can we eliminate stress? What can we do to decrease the stress that makes us gain the unwanted pounds?
A: Well Angela, exercising is great, as we know! Many people are doing it and eliminating their stress. Reading a good book or developing a wholesome hobby. Try to exercise good people skills and giving fewer attitudes. Many

people are just too hyper in a negative way. Stress less by seeing the glass half full in your life!

Dr. Nelson was brilliant and I learned a lot from him! I have experienced stress in my life, and it definitely resulted in weight gain. I feel that a stable foundation in life can be beneficial to you. I knew someone who was engaged, but wanted to call the wedding off. The more she stressed on what to do, the more weight she would gain. It looked as if she gained over 20 pounds of stress. Stress does not care if you are eating healthy or exercising properly.

My weight loss program is full of useful tips, proper ways to prepare your foods, plus mouthwatering recipes that will leave you feeling energized! Stress and food work hand-in-hand. I have moments when I'm feeling down, and because of my mood, I will crave salty foods. Sweets sometimes come to mind, especially chocolate. You just may be wondering how your favorite foods can help you lose weight. Well did you know that you can still eat some of the same foods, if you prepare them the right way?

I want to transform your negative attitude into a positive one, creating a healthy, lean power-house! I will have you walking slowly pass the mirror instead of speed walking. Take notes and mark the information that sets off an alarm in your head. Make up your mind, and be honest with yourself. Do you like what you see? If not, then keep reading, and learn how to become healthy.

Chapter 2
My Reality Check and What I Did About It

You now know what you have to do; so get up and make the change. The following list consists of foods that will help you lose weight:

1. Ginger
2. Blueberries
3. Cinnamon
4. Apple cider
5. Lemons
6. Spinach
7. Oats
8. Wheat Grass
9. Apples

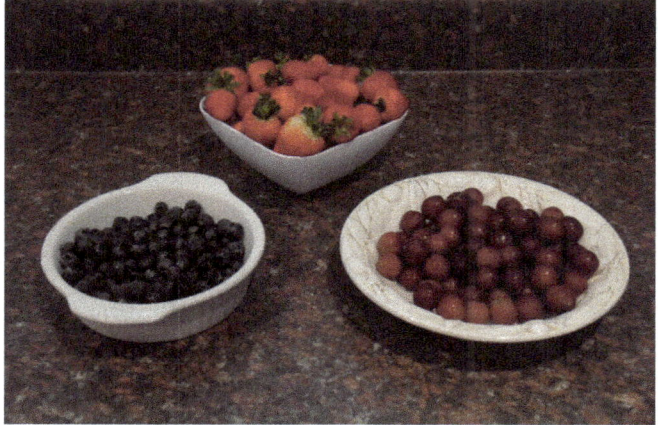

Tip: Try incorporating these foods into your weight loss program, and see how the pounds will come rolling off!

The way in which you prepare your food matters as well. Never eat hot and cold foods at the same time; it causes the digestive system to flow improperly.

- Eat fresh fruit 30 minutes before any solid foods

- Drink warm liquids 30 minutes after you eat solid foods

- Make sure the foods that you eat are room temperature

- In order for your digestive system to flow properly, you have to stop eating two hours before you go to bed

- Every morning and night, drink warm water to allow your foods to digest properly

- Drink green teas without any substitute sugars; instead use one teaspoon of honey (diabetics can use Stevia)

- Jaw Exercise: chew your foods slowly, and it will make you feel full faster

- Keep fresh fruit nearby so that you will not be tempted to eat unhealthy foods

- Start telling yourself that you *can* do this, and believe it in your heart

- Use more herbs and get rid of the high sodium seasonings

- Write out your grocery list before you go shopping, and never shop for food while you are hungry

If you follow these steps, then you can start a successful journey. Eating can be fun, exciting, and full of energy, you just have to choose your path.

When I looked back at some old pictures of myself, I learned much later that I was transforming into an unhealthy, obese woman. My face was always swollen and full of fluid; I began to get depressed. People always considered me the life of the party, but all of a sudden I had retired due to my poor diet. I used to love taking pictures, but all of a sudden I was running from the sound of "say cheese;" instead I ate the cheese! Yes, cheese was and is my addiction. I would run from it, but I would always return to it.

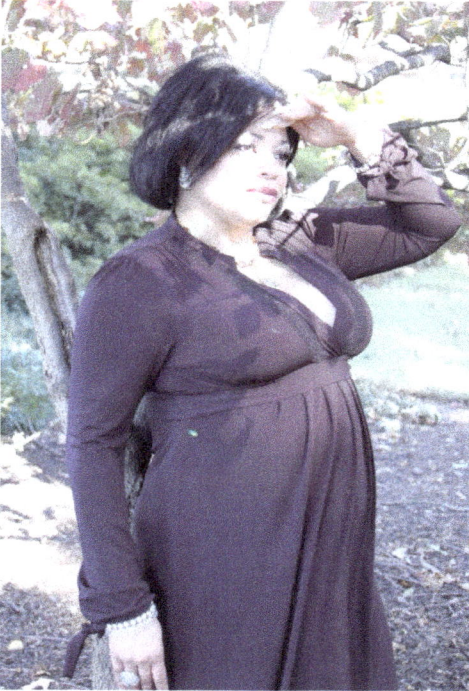

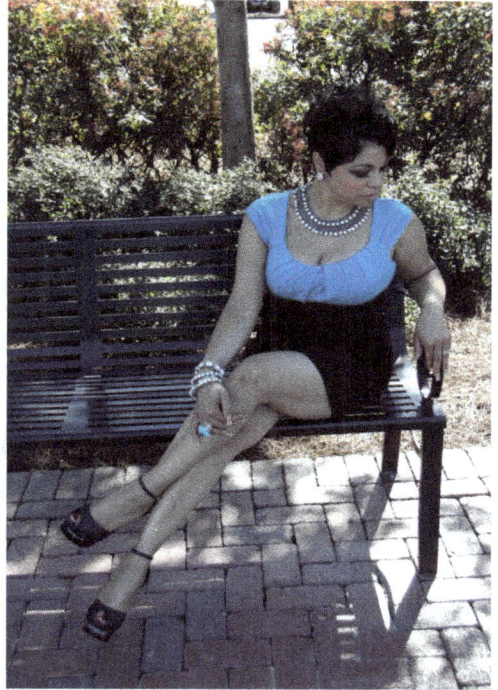

Denial is a terrible thing, but when my physician told me to lose weight, I had to listen. Life has its way of waking you up. I of course was borderline diabetic, and my clothes were moving up in size, and I was wearing the shameful "granny panties!" I became so self-conscious to where my husband would be laughing at the comics in the newspaper, but I would think that he was actually laughing at me. Of course he wasn't, it was just me imagining things. I was quickly losing myself.

I remember waking up and looking in the mirror, and saying, "This is my last day of being FAT!" As brutal as it may sound, I had to be honest with myself. I fell to my knees and prayed to my God to stand and deliver my brand new body. Prayer definitely changes things, but prayer without works is dead (James 2: 20).

My beautiful cousin Tameka blessed me with a book that encouraged me. I was taught so much and it literally changed my life. I was inspired to make extreme changes immediately. My life was about to move into a new and improved transformation. Everyone has their own body mass make up, and you have to be very reasonable about how much weight you should lose or gain.

Going to the department stores was a major headache - I could not fit *anything*. I was literally sweating and complaining about the buyers for the clothes; it was everyone but me. Yes, I had it very bad. I decided that I'd had enough; there was a fine supermodel inside of me and I was determined to show her off! Now motivate yourself with something similar, and make your mind up today.

I had to share my secret, because everywhere I went, I saw obese and over-weight people. I would want to stop them and educate them on what they were doing to their body. Most people, especially women, carry their weight in their abdomen; that is where all the disease and stress lives. Everyday we settle and keep all of our frustrations on the inside. Men and women both stress about relationships, but men are more stressed about their job (finances), and women are more stressed about their children.

The world has developed many stressful issues involving the economy. In the years 2008-2012, many people lost their jobs, homes, and independence. These types of issues ignite the burden of stress, and many people begin to eat in hope that they will forget, and kill the depression.

What I have learned is that now that things are beginning to turn around for people, they are willing to rebuild their hope again!

Chapter 3
The Twenty Day Rule/ A Reflection of Yourself

I'm sure you are wondering what a "twenty day rule" is. The twenty day rule is simply you changing your eating habits. Eating a certain way over a period of time is nothing more than a habit. Plan a trip to your Whole Foods store or local grocery store. Take your time and be patient, because your killer foods will be there, so you must stay focused. There are a number of reasons why people decide to eat bad foods:

- Bored
- Too lazy to cook
- A matter of convenience
- Stressed
- Traveling
- Cheap
- Working over time, and need the salt to stay focused
- Friends and family eat hardy so you eat just as hardy
- You just heard some bad news, and life just got a little hard

Moody Eaters:

- I don't feel like cooking
- The pots I need are dirty
- I am tired and sleepy, and I need it quick
- Fast food is more appealing
- It's the weekend and I want to go out to eat

- I broke up with my significant other, so I am going to eat my blues away
- I just lost my job
- I am failing in college

Under the twenty day rule, remember not to announce to anyone that you're making a life change. People will start to tempt you with food, and this will give you a major setback. Be sure to take a full body picture of yourself, and record your weight. This will serve as a reminder of how you used to look.

Take a look at my tips on breakfast food and noon day snacks.

Breakfast to go Wrap!

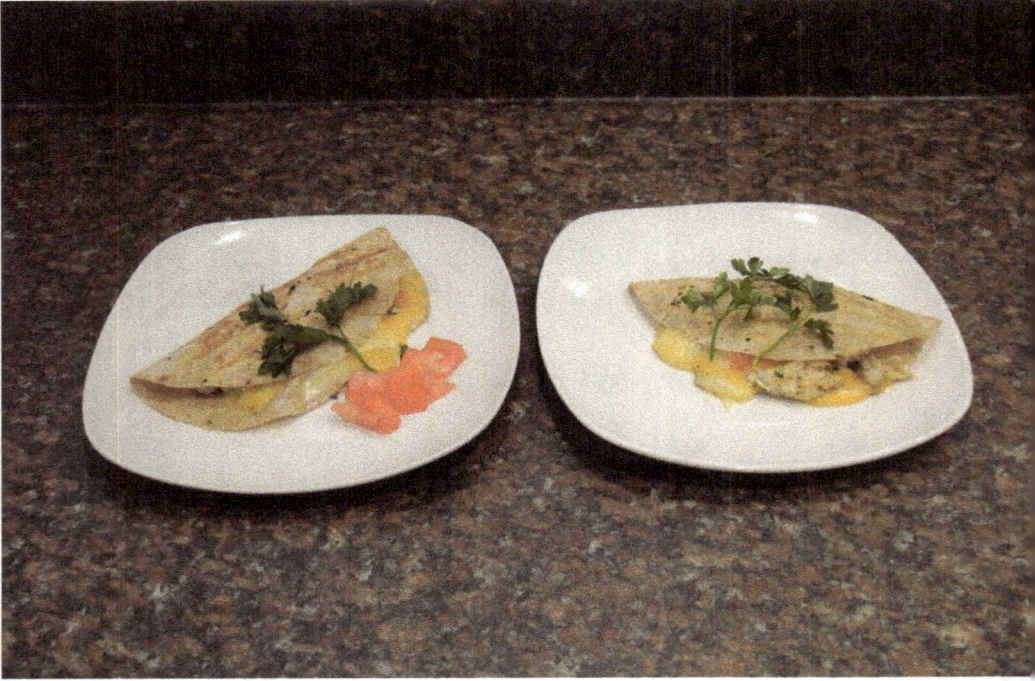

- One large no yoke egg (egg white) scrambled to your desire
- 1/2 cup diced fine tomato
- 1/3 cup of grated 2% cheese with low sodium
- 1/4 cup of chopped mushroom
- One eight ounce grilled chicken breast
- Slice chicken breast in to strips
- Place all ingredients into a 85 gram whole wheat tortilla
- Cook on the griddle with olive oil light
- Allow to brown as desired and enjoy!

Oat Meal with Glazed Apples!

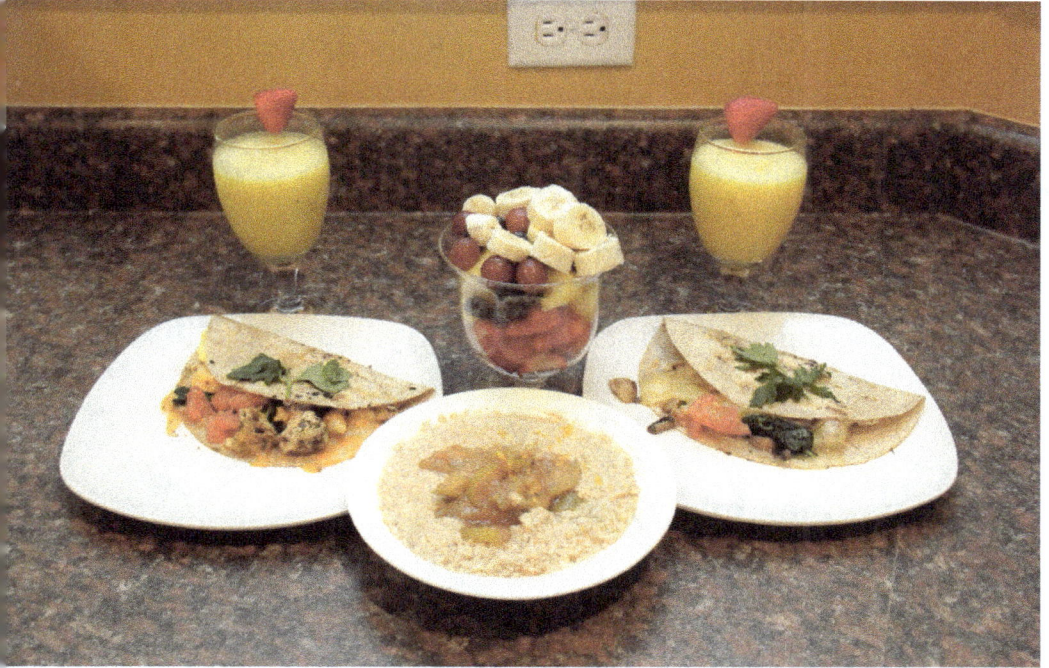

- Boil one cup of water
- Pour one cup of oat meal into a bowl
- Slice two green apples
- Pour apples into a medium sauce pan
- Add 1/2 cup of water
- Add four tablespoons of organic sugar
- Add one teaspoon of cinnamon to boiling water
- Add two tablespoons of unsalted butter to boiling water
- Add 3/4 cup of olive oil light to apples
- Mix

- Add two tablespoons of concentrated lemon juice to keep apple from turning brown
- Bring apples to a soft texture and glaze
- Mix the boiling water into the oatmeal bowl and stir
- Place the glazed apples in the center of bowl and enjoy!

Sometimes you need a delicious juice to get all of your vitamins for the day. This is a terrific juice you will love, and if you are having a breakfast brunch, then your guests will keep coming back for more!

Frozen Pineapple Treat!

- Pour one cup of low sodium orange juice into blender
- Chop chunks of fresh pineapples
- Slice two kiwi
- Slice a half of mango
- Squeeze one fresh lemon into the blender
- Pour all of your ingredients into blender
- Add crushed ice and blend

Now you need some fresh fruit for your guest.

Fresh Fruit Salad!

- Slice strawberries
- Cut chunks of pineapple
- Add blueberries

- Add grapes
- Mix together and place in refrigerator until ready to serve

A Taste of Apple and Cinnamon Pastry!

Now that you have some left over apples, let me show you how to make a hot apple caramel wrap. This is a delicious pastry that your guests will love! You can use peaches, blueberries, apples, or blackberries. It's fruit, therefore it's natural, it's healthy, and it's fun! Oh, don't let me forget to mention that it is **guilt-free**.

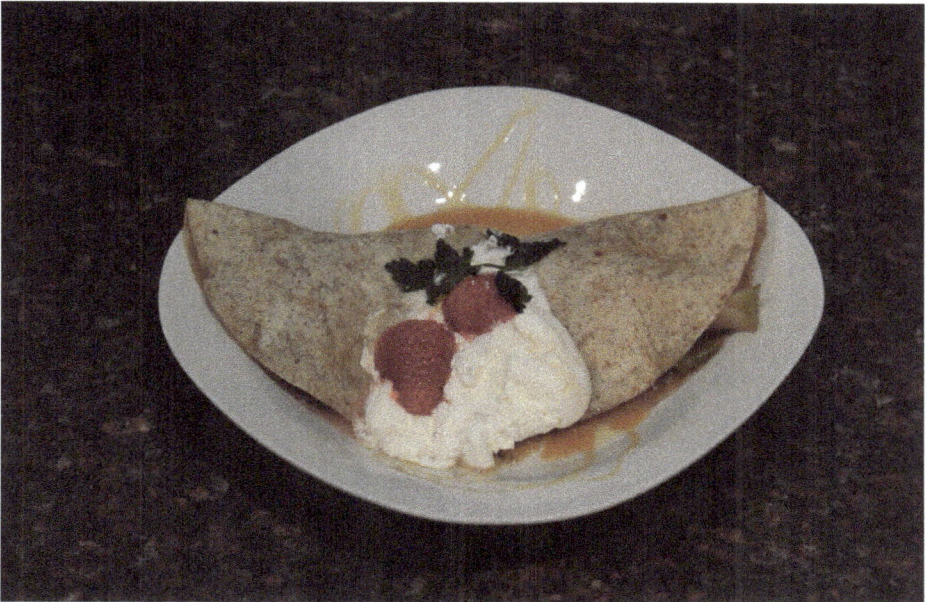

- Preheat oven to 350 degrees
- Place the left over baked apples into a low sodium tortilla
- Seal it by brushing unsalted melted butter around the edges and pinching it shut

- Brush the same melted butter on top
- Place in oven for approximately 10 minutes or until golden brown
- Allow five minutes to cool
- Add fructose free, sugar-free whipped cream on top
- Drizzle 1/2 teaspoon of caramel on top as well.

I would suggest placing your pastry in the center of a dessert plate for added décor.

Now you can enjoy dessert without the guilt!

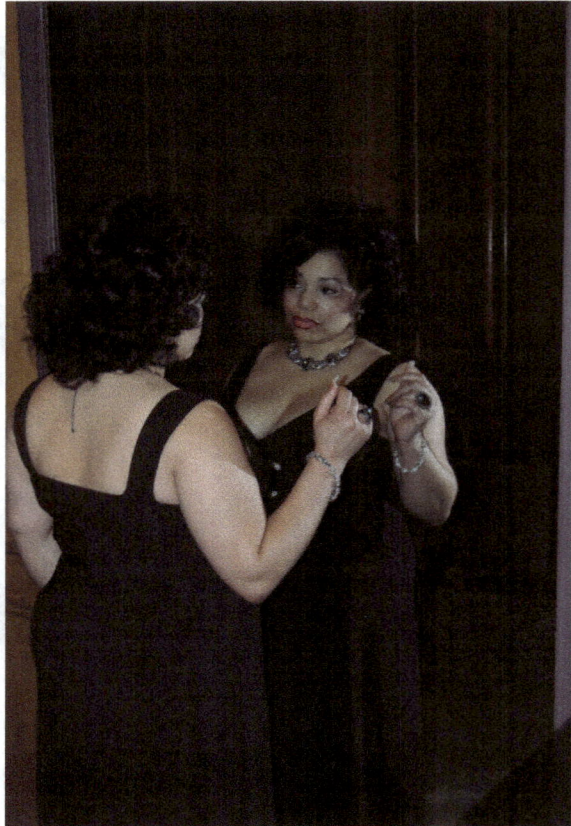

I love to entertain, and give my guests an experience that they will never forget. You can prepare these foods and be sure that they will not have you thinking about a diet!

Sometimes when you're at work or at home, you may become bored, and this can result in you gaining weight. So I have invented some fun snacks that will have you wanting more. Boredom is like a silent whisper in your ear. I have heard it numerous times, playing a horrible tune in my ear. It would tell me,

"Angela, just come into the kitchen and eat some ice cream, potato chips left over pizza, and pound cake."

I had a seven year secret. While my husband would be sleeping I would be eating. One day my secret came out as I began to gain enough weight to make my clothes snug and uncomfortable. Once this happened, the stress came like a thief in the night. So I urge you and encourage you to have these snacks around and make some changes.

Blue Chip Seafood Dip

- Dice four ounces of cooked shrimp
- Lightly season shrimp with tarragon, basil, ginger, Mrs. Dash chicken seasoning, and pepper
- Boil five ounces of fresh crab meat and four ounces of lobster 10-15mins
- Mix all the seafood into a bowl
- Add 1/2 teaspoon of unprocessed organic sugar
- Add chopped parsley
- Add diced sun dried tomatoes
- Add one tablespoon of olive oil light
- Splash a little lime juice over the dip
- Chill in fridge for one hour

You may eat the seafood dip with gluten-free blue chips, and for lower sodium, purchase salt free (it will only be 10 grams of sodium).

A Taste of Winter

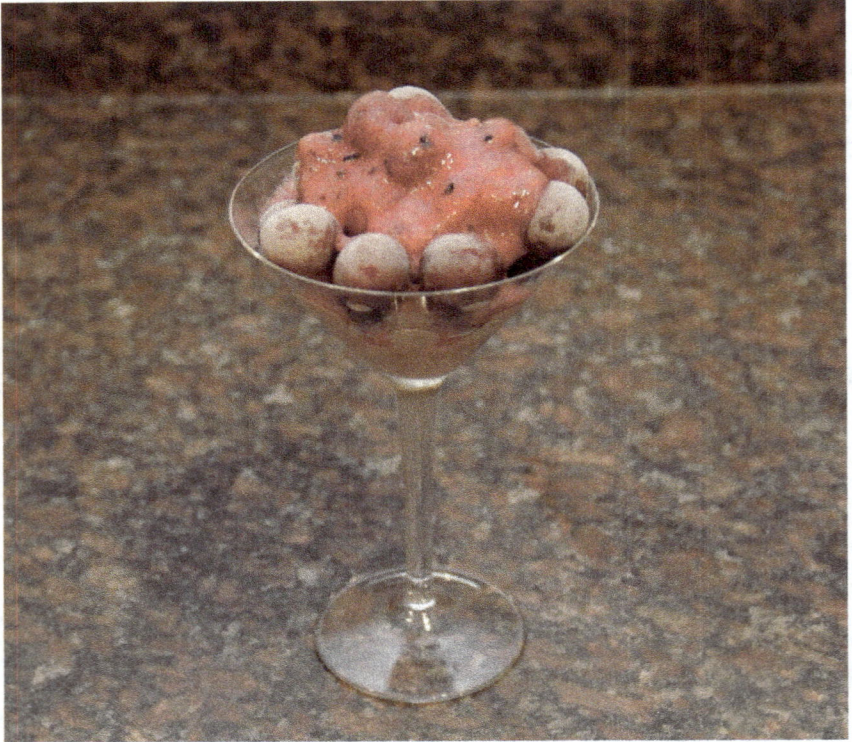

- Clean 13 red seedless grapes
- Place grapes in a bowl
- Cut a whole sweet orange and squeeze on top of grapes
- Place grapes in freezer for one hour

As you indulge in this frosty treat, remember to do your jaw exercises.

These recipes will make your mouth water, and give you an idea of the natural, unprocessed foods that will take you through the twenty day rule. The first rule is to pray, because you may get weak and revert to old habits. Listen to that inner Spirit who is begging you to change right now. Clean out your kitchen, and get ready for war! Your friends, family, and coworkers will test you, so be prepared. It is your time to breathe. Be patient.

Tip: Remember that once you release the stress, then the rest falls into place!

Chapter 4
The Grocery Store (The Crack House)

While going through your twenty day rule, your trip to the grocery store will be like going to the crack house. I have gone down the aisles of the grocery store, and I would literally be shaking, because I was so nervous. I would go down the cookie aisle and reach for the double chocolate chip cookies, but I would draw back. Then I would return in less than five minutes to read how many grams of fat I would actually take in per cookie. If I was stressed I would buy them and eat four cookies on my way home. It wasn't my fault; it was all of the red lights!

Super markets hire workers to sample their foods to customers. Most of these foods are going to be high in fat and sodium. Although this may be a good marketing technique for the grocery store, it is not good for you, because it will lead you to over shop. Many people go to super markets and become impulsive buyers. I used to be gullible and allow people to talk me into buying things that I did not need. We shop, eat, and buy

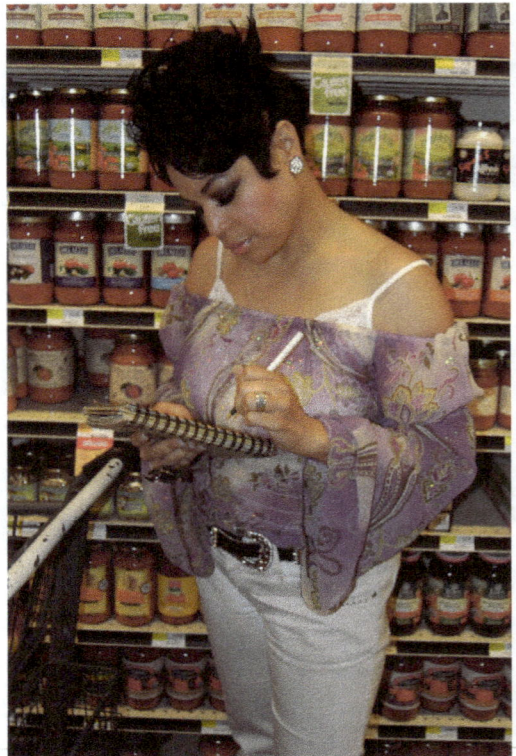

simply because the opportunity presents itself.

When you go to the grocery store, make sure you write out a list of items, and stick-to-your-budget. I have had plenty of budgets, but my total would always turn out to be double what I had planned to spend. I would look in my basket and ask myself, "What did I buy?" The total made me turn red, but I swiped my debit card anyway. When I would get home, I would have so many empty carbs, and items that were high in fat. Most of the foods ranged from 600 – 1200 grams of sodium. I had to eat it or else I would be wasting my food.

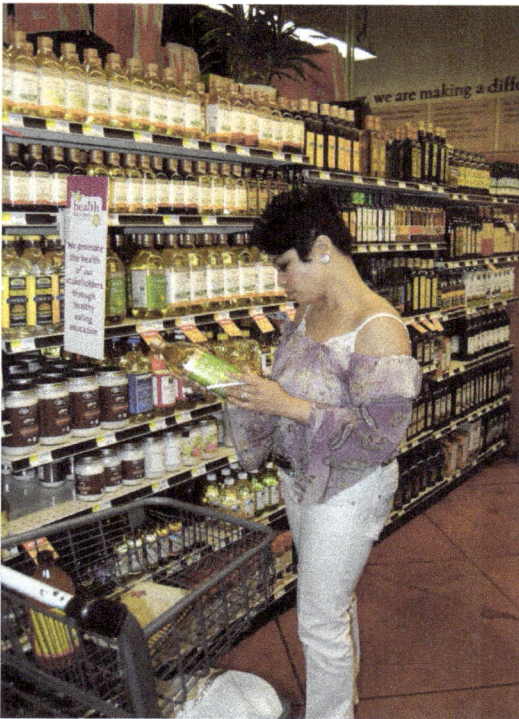

I remember when I was a little girl, my parents would tell me to eat all of my food, because people were starving in Africa. I lived by that for years, and I actually gained a lot of weight from that statement. My advice to you is to eat small portions, and save some for later if you begin to feel full. Your stomach is not as big as you may think it is, so be careful of how much you consume. As you stretch your stomach muscles, the weight begins to enlarge your midsection. I know this because I used to look seven months pregnant! My clients would bump into my stomach and that was *so* embarrassing. The digestive walls are sensitive, so be careful and chew slowly.

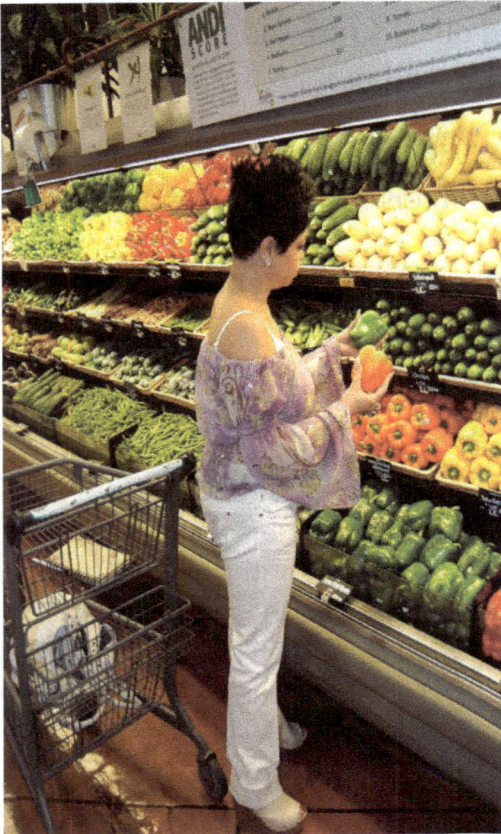

Tip: Eat before you go to the grocery store so that your mind will make more reasonable decisions. Not eating builds up anxiety, and the stressful cravings will start to occur. Also, most cost cutter items need to be ignored, they are never healthy!

Take your time when you first start to shop for healthy foods. Remember to read and know what the ingredients mean. If you have an impatient family member or friend, leave them at home. You need to have a clear understanding of what you are doing. When I first started, I felt lost at the whole foods store. Later I realized that the workers love to help you, and give you advice. It's like being at food school, and they will let you taste the items as well.

Tip: Go online and become an avid reader. Find things that you may like, and try them in a healthy way. What you put in your mouth should matter. Remember, you only have one body. Be honest and get out of the denial phase. Wearing clothes that do not fit is not fixing the problem.

Remember to see your doctor regularly, and when they weigh you, see how your weight is changing. Being over-weight is not the problem; it's not doing anything about it.

Warning signs that you need to change your diet:

- Cancer cells
- Diabetes
- High blood pressure
- High or low cholesterol
- Weight loss or weight gain
- Depression
- Stress
- IBS (Irritable Bowel Syndrome)
- Stiff joints (Arthritis)
- Hair loss or dry scalp
- Heart disease

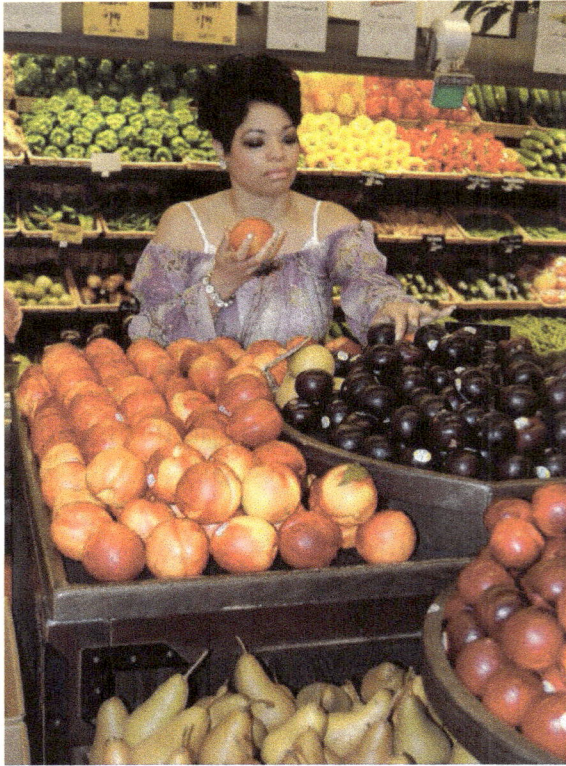

Tip: Take your time and make your trip to the grocery store fun! Read and taste, but be careful. Once you start changing your diet, become more aware of what you are putting into your mouth. You only have one body, and that should mean that you value it and only want to put the very best into it.

The following is what you should look for when you read labels:

- Fructose free products
- Low sodium
- Gluten free
- Low carbs
- Low sugar
- Low fat
- Organic
- Whole wheat

Avoid all foods that have been canned or processed. Avoid starchy items; they are high in sugar and sodium. Avoid juices that are not 100% juice.

Nutrition Facts

Serving Size 1 cup (228g)
Servings Per Container 2

CALORIES

The total calories and calories from fat in one serving.

NUTRIENTS

The metric amounts of fats, cholesterol, sodium, carbohydrate, fiber and protein in one label serving. Sometimes other nutrients are included.

VITAMINS AND MINERALS

The % Daily Value of the vitamins and minerals.

Amount Per Serving

Calories 250	Calories from Fat 110
	% Daily Value*
Total Fat 12g	18%
Saturated Fat 3g	15%
Trans Fat 3g	
Cholesterol 30mg	10%
Sodium 470mg	20%
Potassium 700mg	20%
Total Carbohydrate 31g	10%
Dietary Fiber 0g	0%
Sugars 5g	
Protein 5g	
Vitamin A	4%
Vitamin C	2%
Calcium	20%
Iron	4%

* Percent Daily Values are based on a 2,000 calorie diet. Your Daily Values may be higher or lower depending on your calorie needs.

	Calories:	2,000	2,500
Total Fat	Less than	65g	80g
Sat Fat	Less than	20g	25g
Cholesterol	Less than	300mg	300mg
Sodium	Less than	2,400mg	2,400mg
Total Carbohydrate		300g	375g
Dietary Fiber		25g	30g

*Nutrition Facts label information from *Food, Nutrition & Wellness* by Roberta Duyff, Woodland Hills, CA: Glencoe/McGraw-Hill, 2010

% DAILY VALUE

The percentage that one serving provides of the Daily Value for some nutrients. The % Daily Value also helps you judge how much of a nutrient a serving provides. In the 5-20 guide, 5 percent or less is low; 20 percent or more is high.

PERCENT DAILY VALUES EXPLANATION

Daily Values are based on a 2,000-calorie diet. Your daily value may be higher or lower depending on your calorie needs.

http://www.mealtime.org/uploadedImages/Mealtime/Content/Nutrition%20Facts%20Label(1).jpg

Make sure you understand that the grocery store will be a great life changing experience. Enjoy it and try not to look at it as a chore. If you think negative, then you get those kinds of results. I hope you find something positive and stick to it!

Chapter 5
How Stress Kills Your New Life Style

A lot of the time we exercise and eat right, but the weight doesn't seem to come off as fast as we put it on. The pressure of your life can make you feel like a failure. You need to pray as soon as you wake up and ask God to order all your steps. I did not see any improvements in my life until I let go and let God take care of my enemies. God doesn't need any help from us!

I can laugh now because I know that food comforted me until I laid down my sword, and stopped fighting. I love the way I think and feel now! I went to a health fair and I remember a Life Coach saying that in order to make your life more relaxed, you must do these things:

- Never take calls from negative people when you're tired or stressed
- Choose your battles carefully
- Get a massage on the regular or when you are stressing
- Focus on things that you can change
- When you get off work, relax before you read mail, or solve other people's problems
- Take a short vacation from time to time
- Laugh, because it is the best medicine for the soul
- Indulge in candle light, bubble baths and play soft music
- Pour yourself a glass of red wine and unwind
- Fix yourself a cup of green tea with lemon

Task: Pour yourself a cup of warm green tea with lemon, and nestle into your bed as you read this chapter. I hope you are wearing your best PJ'S, because you just might have to have an intervention.

Sometimes you have to do the very best *you* can do. People will always pull you in different directions. Distractions can cause us to falter. I used to let so many people use me and I was left feeling empty. If God wants me to bless people then I will be obedient. Life is too short to allow dysfunctional people to ruin your life. Some of us allow the minutest thing to take us to a level of high stress.

There are so many things that could stress anyone out. Many times people shop, eat and become mentally depressed from going broke. When you're losing money and running through your 401 K, checking's and savings account, you may run into a wall. Purchasing more expensive foods may be a problem for you. You have to make your dollars stretch, so when you see the discounts and coupons, leap for it! You may start to leave the social life, and start downsizing your entertainment. I too have been there. Every so often, when the stress kicked in, I ate to cope with the problem. I could not see my way out, so I ate doughnuts, pizza, melted chocolate chip cookies, honey gold wings, and much more. It was my short-term fix.

I had a lifestyle where I was able to shop until I dropped. I, along with the good Lord, got that monkey off my back, so to speak. All you need to do is focus on the debt and consider the snowball effect. Start with the small bills and work your way to the monster bills. Breathe, because nothing lasts forever; this too will pass. Life is too short to focus on the negative. Do what you have to do in order to make your situation make sense, but stop eating fatty foods; they only stress you out more. Foods that are high in cholesterol, calories, and sodium, can cause mood swings. So fight your way back to the top, and remember: you can do all things through Christ who strengthens you (Philippians 4:13)!

Most women stress about finding true love, so that causes them to eat and worry all at the same time. There are women who are married with children and the flame has died in their marriage. You just might suspect your spouse to be cheating on you. Many people marry for the wrong reasons, so it won't be long before the drama occurs. I remember I wanted an old boyfriend to be my husband; I was young and passionate about my feelings. He was not my soul mate and I was so blessed that God did not bless that mess. God blessed me with my husband, and we are soul mates.

When you choose and don't pay attention to all the red flags, then you are looking for your airplane to crash. Men and women both can make life changing decisions that have negative results, causing them to eat in order to fill that void. Men sometimes become involved with a scornful woman, and it can cause them a tremendous amount of stress. If he has any children with that woman, then he will face problems. That woman will make his life HELL if she still wants him. I have heard of women who find out if the father of their children has a pay raise, and if he does, she will march right down to Child Support Services and demand more money. Neither one of them is happy, which causes life to become a prison sentence!

Sometimes when one loses their job, or career, they have to regroup. Sometimes you might have to down size. That could be both depressing and embarrassing. People all over, between 2006 and 2012, had lost their homes. Foreclosures had occurred and some even committed suicide, because they could not see any way out.

Learn how to rejoice and be happy for others! In my line of business I have heard so many depressing stories about relationships. People settle and live a lie; they become sick in their heart, and pour a generational curse on their children! The children in turn see all the dysfunction and begin to act out.

Signs that your child/children may be acting out:

- Isolating themselves from the family
- Being disrespectful
- Failing grades
- Changing the way they dress
- Wanting to hang out with their friends more
- Trying to manipulate you
- Not wanting to attend church
- Stealing
- Eating disabilities
- Engaging in sexual activity

You may ask: how does this factor into my weight gain? Stress from your children is definitely why the abnormal eating starts. Parents may start stressing out and kids know when there is trouble in the home. They start to blame themselves and may grow up not knowing how to love, or know what true love is, thus beginning a generational curse. You have to learn how to pray it out; being in denial doesn't solve anything. Marry the

Lord and life will not disappoint you, I did, and I no longer have to worry about being perfect.

I sometimes smile for no reason, because I am at peace with myself. I have joy no matter what happens to me-I know the Lord has me! I am now more open-minded. My problem was trying to be "little miss perfect" and the "know it all." I was also trying to have multiple business ideas, but nothing was quite working out for me. The stress was on a fast roll. When you let go and let God, life is good!

Chapter 6
Quick Meals to Die for

You know we live in a microwave world and people want everything very fast! Sometimes when I would get very hungry, I would panic and eat anything. So now I make sure that I have healthy foods around the house, and at my business. Here are a few to add to your list!

Cheesy Seafood Dip!

- 10 ounces of cooked shrimp
- Two cups of steamed spinach
- Chop 1 cup of fresh tomatoes
- Dice 3/4 cup of mushrooms
- Two cups of 2% low-fat Swiss cheese
- Two cups of 2% low-fat cheddar cheese
- One teaspoon of Tarragon
- Four pinches of pepper
- 1/2 teaspoon of basil
- One tablespoon of Mrs. Dash chicken flavor
- Two ounces of chopped garlic
- 3/4 cup of olive oil light
- Place all ingredients into a non-stick sauce pan on medium heat for 10-12mins
- Cool for 10 minutes

You may serve with unsalted blue gluten-free chips.

Grilled Shrimp Salad

- Grill six ounces of shrimp with two tablespoons of olive oil light, tarragon, Mrs. Dash chicken flavor, and garlic
- Place romaine lettuce into a bowl
- Add one chopped apple
- Add one peeled mandarin orange

Salad Dressing:
- Mix 1/4 cup of olive oil, one fresh squeezed lemon and two oranges
- Add 1/2 teaspoon of tarragon, 1 teaspoon of basil, 1/2 of ginger, 1/4 cup of diced cilantro leaves, and 3/4 cup of balsamic vinaigrette

- Add grilled shrimp to salad
- Toss and serve

Stuffed Cornish Hen

- Preheat oven to 350 degrees
- Remove the liver parts from Cornish Hen
- Rinse with warm water
- Massage one teaspoon of melted, unsalted butter on top of the hen
- Season with garlic, basil, mint, Mrs. Dash chicken flavor, tarragon, pepper, and garlic
- Place hen in the center of a greased baking dish

- Bake for 30 minutes
- Grill some colorful bell peppers and oranges, and stuff into the hen
- Bake an additional 10 minutes
- Grill some asparagus in olive oil light, and season lightly, with pinches of tarragon, Mrs. Dash chicken flavor, ginger, garlic, cilantro, and pepper
- Place a sweet potato in microwave for 15 minutes, when done drizzle with one teaspoon of unsalted butter and cinnamon

Enjoy!

This will make a wonderful holiday meal. Remember, you can eat, but say good-bye to the guilt!

Low Fat Chocolate Strawberry Brownie

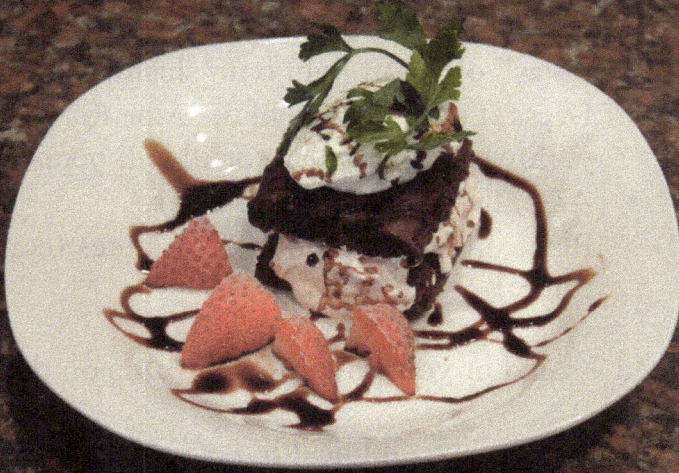

- Cut 15 strawberries and place in a bowl
- Add one 16oz container of sugar free, fructose free whipped cream into the same bowl
- Shave 1/2 teaspoon of orange hull into bowl
- Sprinkle one teaspoon of cinnamon into bowl
- Mix all ingredients
- Place two fiber one brownies on a platter
- Scoop strawberry filling on to one of the brownies and top with the other brownie
- Place in the freezer for 20 minutes

Shrimp Skewer

- Prepare your fresh water unsalted shrimp
- Season lightly with tarragon, pepper, Mrs. Dash chicken flavor, basil, and garlic
- Splash olive oil light onto shrimp
- Dress it up with zucchini, grape tomatoes, yellow squash, and colorful bell peppers
- Add all ingredients to skewer
- Place on grill for ten to 12 minutes (constantly rotate)

You may add a salad or your favorite vegetable on the side.

It's fun, it's tasty, and healthy!

Chicken Skewer

- Prepare an eight ounce piece of skinless chicken breast
- Massage chicken breast with olive oil light
- Season lightly with Mrs. Dash chicken flavor, tarragon, basil, and pepper
- Add grape tomatoes and red bell peppers
- Start building the skewers
- Place on grill (constantly rotate)
  ## Spinach
  - Sprinkle lemon juice onto spinach
  - Season lightly with tarragon, basil, and ginger
  - Mix in two teaspoons of olive oil

Eat as a healthy snack and watch how you will crave this delicious treat all over again!

Fruit Skewer

- Prepare fresh strawberries, red seedless grapes, pineapples, melons, and apples
- Splash lemon juice on apples to keep your color fresh
- Build your skewer

You can use this idea to build your own fruit arrangement, which can be used as a centerpiece. It reminds your guests to eat smart and healthy. More importantly, this idea makes eating more sanitary for multiple people.

Many people have spent thousands of dollars on unnecessary weight loss surgery, but if you're determined to lose weight, then good eating and exercise will aid you in that process. In order for you to make this change, you need to find your inner strength and pray for positive changes; find a nutritionist and educate your self on good eating. Explore your options, and become open to change. I hear people all the time say what they will not consider eating. I was that person, close-minded, and all at the same time borderline diabetic. Take a long look at your health and see if what you're not willing to do makes sense. I love the quote, "You can take a man to the water, but you can't make him drink."

These are some of the things that people hinder themselves from:

- Success
- Business
- New careers
- Relationships
- Higher Education
- Spiritual Growth
- Being in their God given purpose
- Meeting positive networking people
- Having peace and joy
- Eating well and LOVING IT!

It's your turn to make the same decision. Are you willing to drink the "water"? Life is too short to keep procrastinating.

Chapter 7
The Education of Good Eating

I have learned what good food can do for your body. With that said, I want you to try to add something new to your list of foods every so often. Remember to be open-minded and focus on good health. I love going online and researching what my body needs and doesn't need. In my research, I have found the top vegetables that love your body.

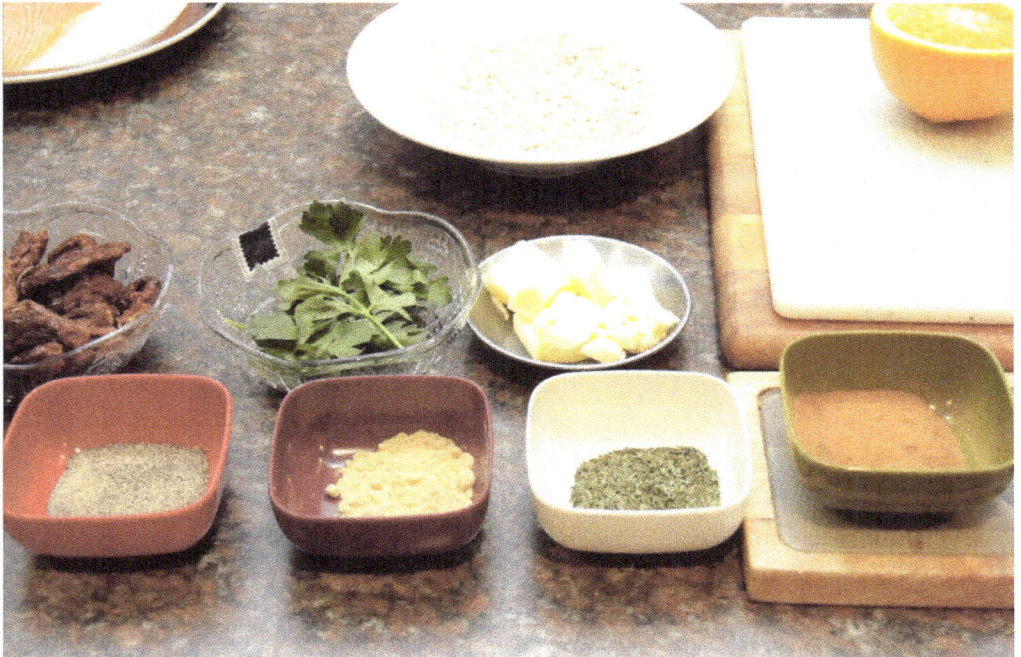

- Spinach is good for obtaining your vitamins, eye health, and memory improvement.

- Broccoli has high levels of antioxidants. Steamed broccoli reduces heart attack by boosting the ability to fight off cell damage.
- Carrots are a source of nutrients; they are incredibly rich in both alpha- carotene and beta carotene, which both convert into vitamin A. They have a *ton* of fiber.
- Zucchini is low in saturated fat and sodium, and is very low in cholesterol. It has a good source of protein, vitamin A, thiamin niacin, phosphorus, and copper; which makes it a good source of dietary fiber, vitamin C, vitamin K, riboflavin foliate, BC, magnesium, potassium, and manganese.

Try mixing and matching fruits and vegetables in these items:

- Soups
- Salads
- Wraps
- Skewers
- Juice
- With your protein meal
- Shakes
- Smoothies

You invent the wheel and make eating more interesting. I once tried spinach and ice cream - it was *so* delicious! My life is changing and I am living a more positive life.

I have found that eating gluten-free foods decreases a lot of irritable bowel syndrome symptoms. Gluten is the protein in wheat, rye, barley, spelt, and a few other closely related grains, however, gluten is not in corn, rice, or oats. Oats are contaminated during processing by the ones that are gluten-free in a gluten-free environment. Many people have experienced wonderful results from maintaining a gluten-free diet.

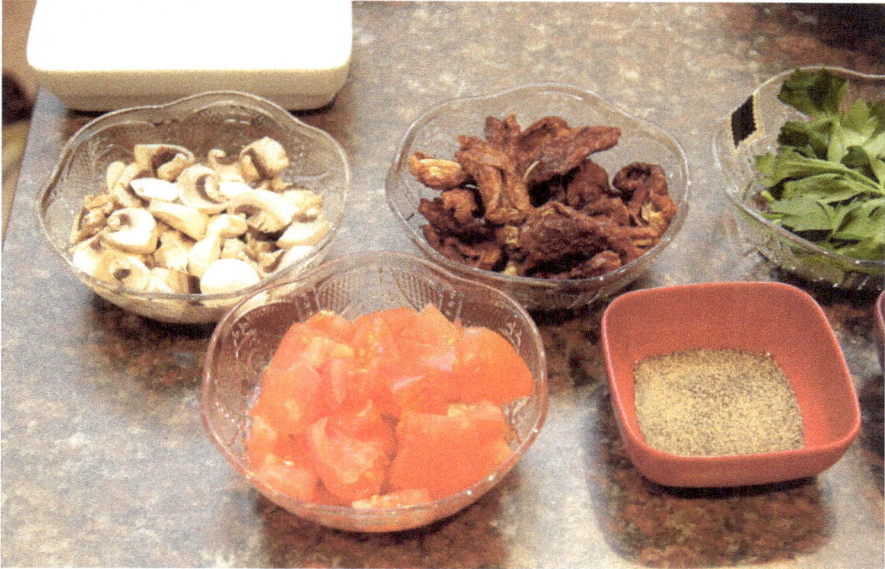

This list contains things that you may discover about maintaining a gluten-free diet:

- A better night's sleep
- Losing weight
- No bloating after eating
- Improved digestive system
- Improved immune system
- Positive attitude

Grains and Baked Foods Containing Gluten

Wheat	Barley	Rye
Bread and Bread Rolls	Rye Bread, Pumpernickel	Yorkshire Pudding
Pretzels	Cakes	Stuffing and Dressings
Muffins	Pastries or Pie Crust	Pancakes
Biscuits or Cookies	Pasta (macaroni, spaghetti, etc.)	Crisp Breads
Bulgur Wheat	Durham	Crumble Toppings
Couscous	Pizza Dough	Semolina
Scones	Batter	Breakfast Cereals
All Bran	Sponge Puddings	Bread Crumbed Ham

Bagels	Cheesecakes	Muesli
Crumpets	Shortbread	Dumplings
Spelt	Triticale	Batter

GLUTEN-FREE VEGETABLES AND FRUITS

Winter	Spring	Summer	Autumn/Fall
Beetroot	Purple Sprouting Broccoli	Asparagus	Wild Mushrooms
Cabbage	Carrots	Courgettes (Zucchini)	Sweet corn
Leeks	Spring onions (Scallions)	Mange Tout	Beetroot

Onions	New potatoes	Globe Artichokes	Sweet corn
Brussels Sprouts	Spring greens	Garden Peas	Cauliflowers
Shallots	Lettuces	Green beans	Carrots
Parsnips	Asparagus	Cucumber	Marrows
Swede	Broad beans	Lettuces	Broccoli
Spinach	Spinach	Radishes	Butternut squash
Curly Kale	Rhubarb	Watercress	Turnips
Artichokes		Peppers	Cabbages
Pumpkin		Tomatoes	Parsnips
Apples		Sweet corn	Celery

Pears

Nuts

Bananas (year round)

Oranges (year round)

Summer berries

Leeks

Cherries

Apples

Currants

Pears

Plums

Almonds

Melons

Chestnuts

Apricots

Elderberries

Grapes

Figs

With this information, will you make the change? All vegetables are gluten-free as long as you avoid adding any gluten foods to them. You may not see yourself divorcing these foods, but if you're gaining weight and becoming stressed out with life, then make the necessary changes. You can be the motivation to those around you by changing your lifestyle.

I often wondered, for many years, why food sometimes made me sick and caused me pain and bloating. I watched my body transform itself, while I became a stranger in my own skin. I always loved myself, but I was lacking knowledge. There are still people who look at my transformation and they still cannot believe the results. I even have to take a second look sometime, and admire what God has done! My faith keeps me strong.

I am in a YES-I-CAN mood; does that statement sound familiar? Get excited about change! I hear so many people complaining about change, but change is good! Once you make healthy eating a lifestyle, and surround yourself with people who are truly committed to the idea, you get results.

I now have a passion for diabetics, because I understand that foods can increase the disease. Eating healthy will give your body a rest. Many people have changed their eating habits and weaned themselves off of medications, because of their improved diet. When you are a diabetic your cells glucose to help your body better function. Glucose gets into the cells when insulin, much like a key, opens the cell up to take in glucose. A person with diabetes does not produce insulin, so the glucose does not get into the cell.

Diabetes often goes undiagnosed because many of its symptoms seem so harmless.

Recent studies indicate that the **early detection** of diabetic symptoms and treatment can decrease the chance of developing the **complications of diabetes**.

If you are experiencing one or more of these symptoms, see your doctor immediately.

Type 1 Diabetes

- Frequent urination
- Unusual thirst
- Extreme hunger
- Unusual weight loss
- Extreme fatigue and Irritability

Type 2 Diabetes

- Any of the type 1 symptoms
- Frequent infections
- Blurred vision
- Cuts/bruises that are slow to heal
- Tingling/numbness in the hands/feet
- Recurring skin, gum, or bladder infections

Gestational Diabetes

- Frequent urination
- Unusual thirst
- Extreme hunger
- Unusual weight loss
- Extreme fatigue and Irritability

Food for Thought: Did you know that there are at least 23.6 million people who have been diagnosed with diabetes and 6 million people are not even aware that they even have diabetes? Over 180,000 people have died, they usually have, heart attacks, strokes, or even kidney failure. There are an estimated 600 million people with diabetes globally. These numbers bothered me deeply, and my passion is to help those who want to get on board and receive valuable information that will keep them alive and well!

Chapter 8
Quick and Easy Meals that Make Sense

Seeing as your knowledge of healthy eating is expanding, you can make your meals more exciting! This chapter will give you some good ideas for parties, as well as snacks, and family dinners. If you are cooking for one or two people, decrease the portions, and save some for later. I am in such high spirits for you! When you are losing weight makes it fun and not a chore. You need to have power over your body and your mind. Change is good! So get up and stop eating that fast-food that will leave your hands greasy and your arteries clogged!

I was parking my car one day and I watched an over-weight woman eat a greasy burger and fries! I used to do that. She looked at me with shame. So I ask you, after you finish eating foods that are high in saturated fat, how do you feel? Do you find yourself feeling guilty, ashamed, or even sluggish? I had no idea I was slowly killing myself and risking, heart-disease, diabetes, stroke, and heart-attacks. Love yourself enough to transform your life into one that is healthy.

These are the types of foods that will continue to hinder you if you don't give them up:

- Cheese burgers
- Pizza
- Hot dogs
- Fried chicken
- French fries
- Cakes
- Ice cream
- Doughnuts

- Chips
- Cookies
- Loaded baked potatoes
- Onion rings
- Pork bacon
- Pancakes
- Biscuits

Tip: Try foods that are healthy, but think outside of the box while you are doing so. Close your eyes and see if you love the foods without looking at the way it appears, that way you aren't judging the taste from what you see.

Imagine yourself on an island and there are only fruits, vegetables, and fresh protein meats. Would you starve to death? I don't think you would. You would adapt to that lifestyle and accept the change. Now that I have set the scene for you, take a look at the mouthwatering recipes that you can add to your list of healthy ideas.

Fresh Fish Taco

- Lightly season an 8 ounce tilapia with tarragon, Mrs. Dash chicken flavor, basil, and ginger
- Sprinkle olive oil light over tilapia
- Spray olive oil on indoor grill to keep from sticking
- Rotate on grill for about 10 minutes
- Remove from grill and set aside for later
- Cut bell peppers and fresh mushrooms
- Lightly spray bell peppers and mushrooms with olive oil light, and place on grill for seven minutes
- Season fresh baby spinach with tarragon, basil, and a pinch of ginger
- Add seasoned spinach to the grill
- Grill spinach for one minute, then remove
- Remove all items from grill and place a whole wheat 85 gram sodium tortilla on grill
- Brush 1/2 teaspoon of unsalted butter on tortilla to keep from sticking
- Place tilapia, spinach, bell peppers, mushrooms, and 2% milk Swiss cheese on tortilla
- Fold wrap down and grill for three minutes

Food for Thought: You can substitute cheese for fruit. Also, slice some melons and tomatoes; add olive oil light and tarragon, basil, and cilantro. Mix it together and add it to the wrap-enjoy!

Orange You Surprised!

Depending on how many people you are expecting:

- Rinse 6-10 sweet oranges
- Cut the bottom of the oranges so they can sit without rolling
- Take a sharp knife and carve out the middle; place the skin of the orange in a bowl for later
- Clean fresh strawberries, blueberries, pineapples, bananas, and kiwi
- Place in a blender along with the pulp of the orange
- Add one cup of 100% juice to the blender
- Place on smoothie and blend
- Pour into the hollow oranges
- Place oranges in the freezer for an hour
- Place a strawberry on the side for decoration, and serve with a spoon

You will be a hit at your dinner party! Warning in advance, your guest will ask you for this recipe. It will be up to you to share. Orange you glad that you are going to be the life of the party?

Tropical Fruit Popsicle

Get fun molds and make it colorful for your children

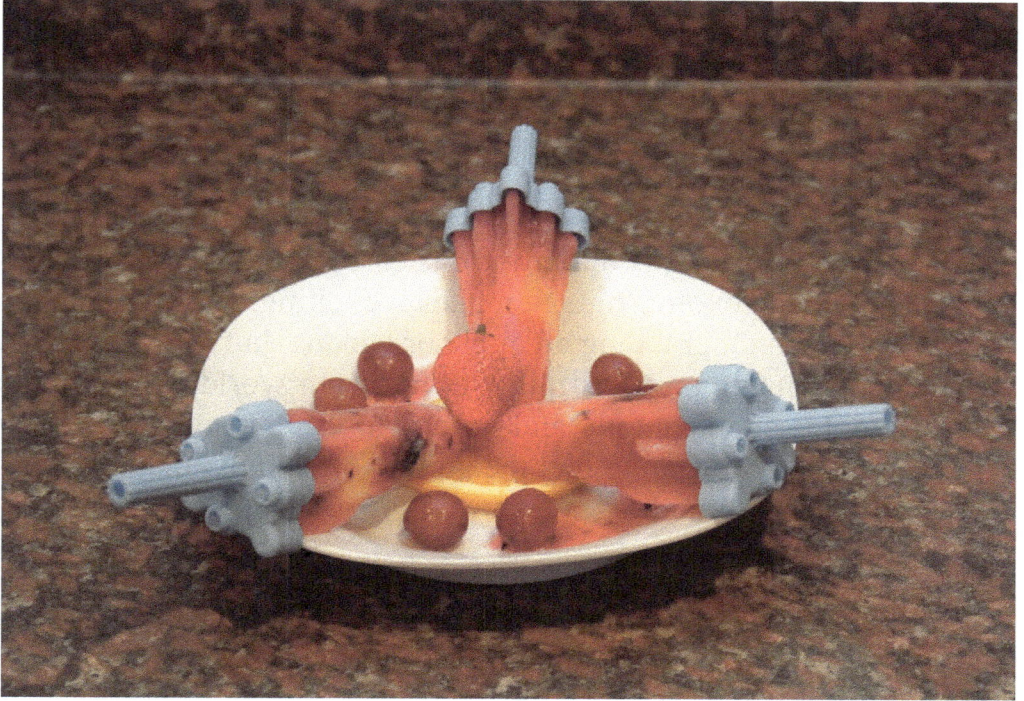

- Prepare fresh strawberries, kiwis, raspberries, blueberries, pineapple, banana, oranges, and mango
- Cut the strawberries, mango, pineapple, banana and kiwis into small chunks
- Pour one cup of Healthy Balance grape juice into blender
- Shave the orange hull into blender for natural sweetness
- Place all fruit into blender and blend on smoothie

- Pour the fruit juice into the molds, and add small chunks of fruit as well
- Place popsicles into the freezer until frozen
- Place popsicle under warm water to loosen mold

This chilled delight will make a great summer treat, and moms, your children can help too! This is a great way for you to reduce your children's sugar in take, while making a memorable experience.

Simply using your daily fruits can be dull and boring, but when you add exotic fruits, it makes it exciting. Usually I would frown on grabbing an apple or banana, but now I *crave* them. When you prepare fruit with fun, your world will begin to change. I used to eat fatty and starchy foods, but soon after I was finished, I began to feel the guilt. Now I know that I'm worthy of good foods!

Better Than Banana Split Surprise
Makes 4-6 servings

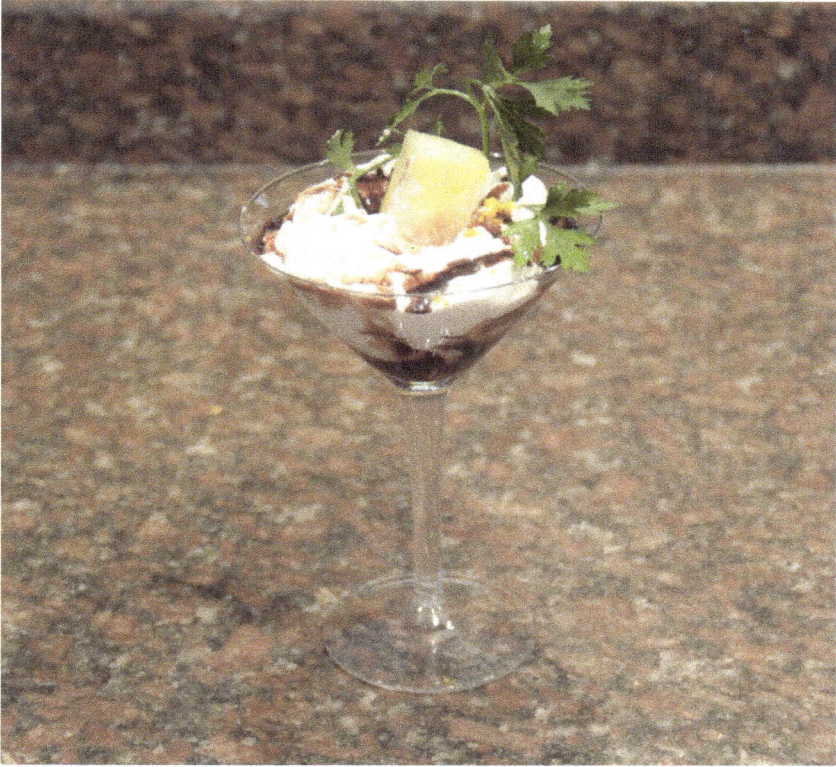

- Cut four bananas and place into a medium bowl
- Add one teaspoon of Stevia sugar into bowl
- Add one large 16oz container of fructose free, sugar free whipped cream into bowl
- Shave 1/2 teaspoon of orange hull into bowl
- Mix all ingredients
- Place bowl into freezer for 20 minutes

Once you key in to the education of good foods, then you have accomplished what you set out to do. Don't worry about slip ups, they will happen, but continue pressing on. If you are serious, then every time you look in the mirror, you will say, "I AM WORTHY OF GOOD HEALTH!" We often get distracted, but remember to get back on the horse and ride out your life journey! If you know who you are, and what your purpose in life is, then you will begin to move into what God has framed for you.

Sometimes when I meet people, it seems that they all want the same thing: good health and to lose weight. I love telling those people my story of how I was them - lost and feeling hopeless. I look in to their soul and I know that I have to share the truth with them. It is my God given purpose to inspire people who are diabetics, over-weight, and stressed out about life. Losing weight is about making your mind up, and transforming your old, bad habits into good habits.

Let's move on with some more recipes that you will crave from time to time!

Juicy Turkey Meatballs

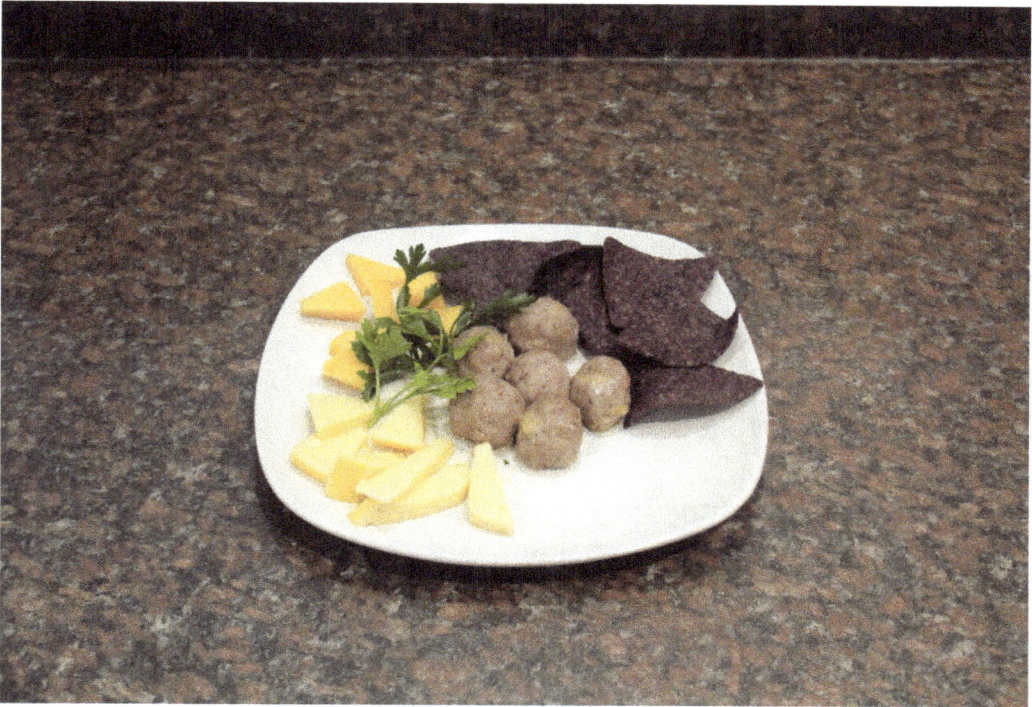

- Preheat oven to 350 degrees
- One pound of fresh ground turkey
- Season lightly with tarragon, Mrs. Dash chicken flavor, pepper, basil, garlic, and ginger
- Massage olive oil light into the turkey meat
- Mix in one cup of shredded 2% Swiss cheese
- Roll turkey meat into balls
- Place meatballs on a baking sheet and cook for 20 minutes
- Remove from oven and serve!

Sweet Cinnamon Baked Potato

- Clean a fresh sweet potato
- Punch holes into the sweet potato using a fork
- Place sweet potato on a microwavable plate and place in the microwave
- Heat on potato
- Cut sweet potato open
- Add one teaspoon of cinnamon
- Add one teaspoon of unsalted butter
- Sprinkle with 1/2 teaspoon of organic unprocessed sugar
- Mix it together and enjoy!

This is a healthy way to eat your sweet potato, and it is far healthier than the white potato. You can eat this instead of candied yams, because it has less sugar and butter, and your waistline will love you for ever!

I love tasting vegetables, fruits, and meats before fatty ingredients ruin the experience. I remember going to an upscale restaurant where they poured so much salt on my shrimp that I couldn't even enjoy it! I was paying for fresh shrimp, but the salt destroyed my desire for the sea food altogether. I used to over season my foods, but after I discovered that I was gaining weight from the sodium, I decided that "less is more." Now I'm conscious when people invite me over to eat, because when you start changing your food intake, your body might reject pork, beef, salt, pasta, or sugar.

Here are some more great ideas that will expand your list of recipes, and help you continue this journey!

Grilled Salmon and Chips

Go to your fresh fish market and buy a salmon to feed a dinner party of eight.

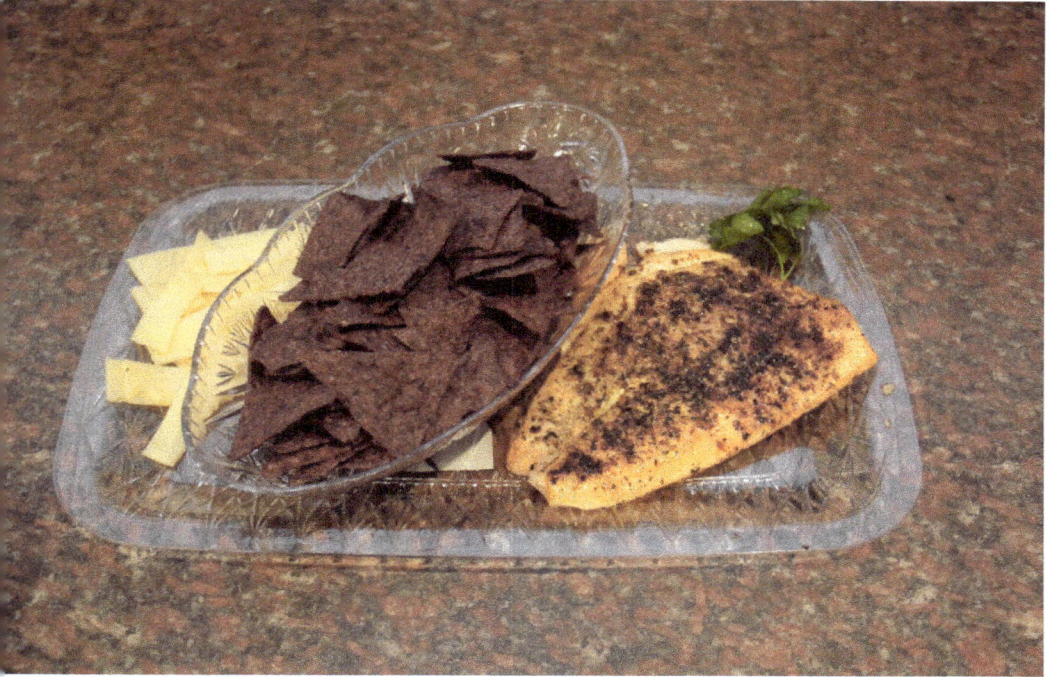

- Season your salmon lightly with tarragon, basil, ginger, Mrs. Dash chicken flavor, and garlic
- Massage olive oil on top
- Place on grill until light pink or until well done
- Grill oranges and lemons
- Place grilled oranges and lemons on the grilled salmon

Dress up your platter with unsalted gluten-free blue chips and place the salmon in the center of the platter. Cut some Swiss cheese and place on the other side of platter.

This is a healthy hors d'oeuvre for your guest, and they will never think of it as being diet food. Simple dishes are much better than over the top, fattening ones. Your dinner parties can be a healthy success; you just have to reinvent the wheel. People often ask me what they should eat next. I tell them to read my book and your world will change! I do not promote not eating; I just give people better eating options that have helped me and others. I used to have to loosen my clothes in order to enjoy a good meal, but now I don't. My body no longer rejects the food I eat; instead, it loves the foods that I eat.

Burn Baby Burn

- Pour two ounces of apple cider vinegar into a coffee mug
- Add two ounces of concentrated lemon juice
- Fill the rest of the coffee mug with a low sugar juice
- Stir, and sip slowly for 30 minutes

The benefit is that it lowers your high blood-pressure, and it burns off the fat, making you look and feel young again!

Chapter 9
Where Did All of My Stress Go: An Interview with Deana Taylor

When you start eating better, and including exercise in to the equation, then you have made it. Although I was able to lose 55 pounds without exercise, I still needed energy and fuel. Your heart needs that strong muscle to help you stay healthy. I had the opportunity of speaking with someone who encouraged me to exercise and firm up my body - Deana Taylor. Deana Taylor has a Bachelor's of Science Degree in Biology from the University Of Memphis, and is the owner of Finally Fit Memphis. I had the pleasure of asking her a host of questions about exercise and healthy eating.

Q: Deana, were you ever over weight?
A: Yes, when I had my son. I was 130lbs and after I gave birth I was 187 pounds.

Q: How did you begin losing the weight?
A: I made my mind up. I kept a journal and I did a strategy on how I would work out. If you can conquer the

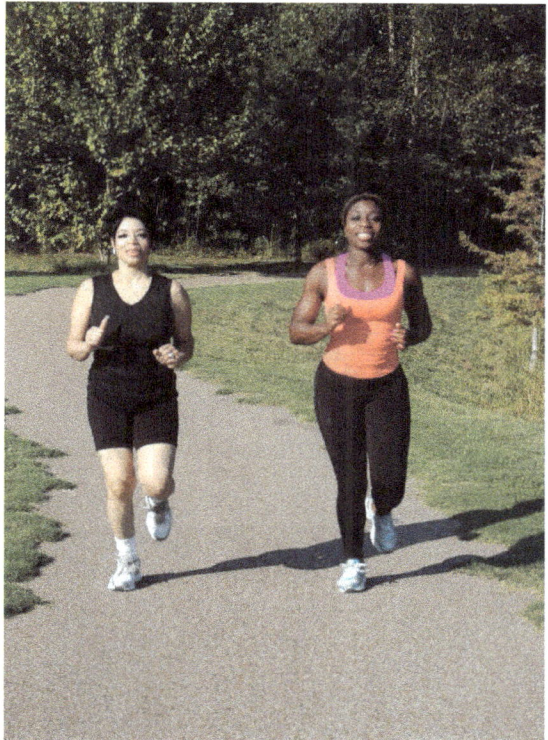

mind, you have made it!

Q: As a beginner, what should someone do to get started, without hurting themself?
A: Light walking or jogging, or a beginner's class. Build up strength with light push-ups, light weight training, and cardio exercises.

Q: When exercising, is it better to go to the gym or to get a personal trainer?
A: A personal trainer would be better, so you can know how to use the equipment, and to know your limitations. Also, you can get a one-on-one experience! You should target towards what you really need to concentrate on. A personal trainer could be that road map!

Q: Should you consult a physician before you exercise?
A: Definitely, because you may get light headed, and you may not be able to do all of the things listed on the program. You need to check your heart level, and if you're a diabetic, you really need a release form from your physician. I have had a client who did not consult his physician and he passed out!

Q: Should you eat healthy while working out?
A: Yes, because you should not put junk on top of exercising - it defeats the purpose. You will get very little results. You get internal issues like colon cancer, heart disease, diabetes, and other high risk issues as well, if you aren't eating properly!

Q: What can I do at home if I have no time and I am on a budget? **A:** The best is cardio, strength training, lifting light weights, 15 jumps, push-ups, and crunches and repeat it three sets. Make sure you do abdomen work in sets of threes every morning and night!

Q: Should someone consume alcohol while trying to lose weight? **A:** You should use moderation, and be careful of what kind of alcohol you are drinking.

Q: What are the positive results for getting rid of stress, and what techniques can help along the way? **A:** Breathing techniques work, being positive, and feeling that you are doing something good. Pilates and yoga works as well, as for eliminating stress. Your body will respond to moving all of your muscles that you may not have moved in years.

Q: How should one warm-up before exercising? **A:** Two different types: static and dynamic stretching.

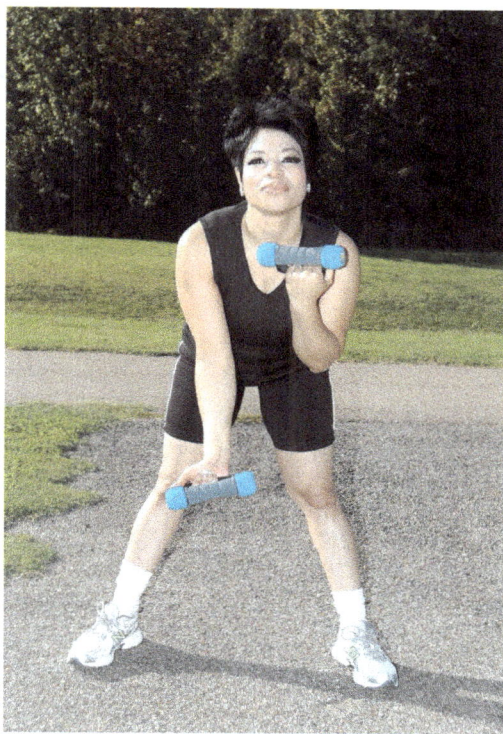

- Static is about holding muscles in place, or holding the position in place. Like reaching and touching your toes.
- Dynamic is more of a continued touching (more movements.) Running in place, lunges, shoulder-rolls forward, and shoulder-rolls backward. Pilates and yoga exercises. Also sitting and reaching.

Q: After someone has lost the weight, and then begins to regain it, what should they do mentally and physically to get back on the right track?
A: They need to go back and create a work out plan that works for their schedule. Get back on board with a nutritionist, retract what got them off track, and try to keep from doing it all over again.

For more information please contact Deana Taylor, so that you can be on top of your game!

I hope now you understand how good eating and exercise work. Remember, take it slow. Once you have had a good work out, eat a salad and eat some fruit, or make a smoothie. Have a dinner that is full of protein, and drink warm water right before you go to bed, to loosen the food in your stomach. You can add a lime or lemon to burn calories. In the morning repeat the same process.

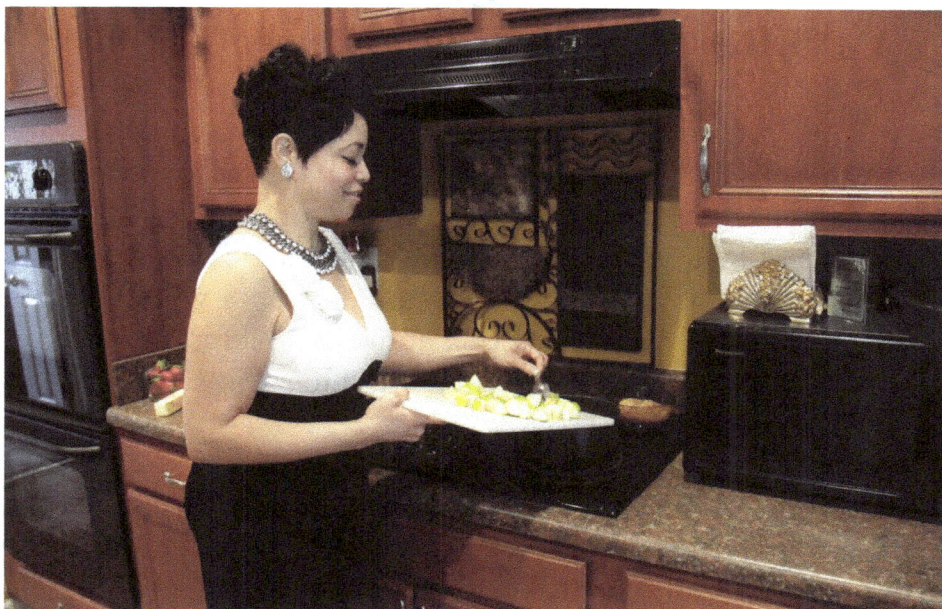

     While working out and eating healthy, do a monthly cleansing to keep your body healthy and disease free. Keep your preparation time for your meals under 30 minutes, simply delicious and health conscious. Never compromise your new healthy life experience! You will transform yourself into the new 80 instead of that old 20. This means you will be up graded and sitting on a high white horse! People will begin to ask you what you're doing. Do not forget to give back and let them know how you got there. Pray every day to remain on track. Remember: you are human and you make mistakes, but with God on your side, all things will work in your favor. Amen!

Chapter 10
I Have Made It and I'm Loving The NEW Me

Now that you understand how healthy eating plays a vital role in your life, you can move forward. Being over-weight occurs when we are not eating properly, or exercising, and because of that, we start shying away from the world and become in denial about our weight. For years I would look in the mirror, but I would not look at the real picture. People see what they want to see, becoming blind to reality.

On the other hand, there are a lot of under-weight people, or people who have a high metabolism. These people still need to eat properly, because they are not exempt from disease, heart-attack, stroke, diabetes, cancer, or anything else that may harm their health. We have to be healthy inside and out in order to achieve total wellness.

When you're a diabetic, cheating on your new life style only causes serious problems with your higher blood sugar levels. It may also cause you to have long-term health problems. Work with your physician to develop a disease management plan. Your disease management plan should include:

- Diet: what to eat, when to eat it, and how much to eat
- Exercise: types of exercise, workout schedule, desired pre- and post-workout glucose levels. Always keep a snack with you in case your blood sugar drops too low. Always listen to your body, and alert a personal trainer of your medical condition.
- Medication: type, dosage, when to take it, how to store it.

- Medical care: wear a patient ID bracelet; provide your workplace and gym with your physician's contact information.
- Goals(what you want to achieve): whether it's preventing diabetes, managing it or getting off insulin

Remember, you can have a healthy life-style; you just have to manage your body. Many people give up and continue in their unhealthy eating habits because they may:

- Feel like giving up
- Feel depressed
- Feel lost and don't understand the disease
- Be stubborn, and feel like they will eventually die from something
- Love eating fatty foods and will not give it up
- Be that their environment doesn't permit them to change
- Live a very busy life and will not stop to make the necessary changes

If this is you, then please make the best decision of your life and change. Prayer changes things. I know this because I have made so many mistakes without prayer. THE POWER OF PRAYER CHANGES THINGS!

You can transform your way of thinking by simply knowing about your mind, body, and soul. Allow your thoughts to become pure, and you will become whole. Educate yourself on how stress affects your body. If you have a disease, research the symptoms and try new, inspiring ways to improve the situation. As you begin to lose your stress and weight, start a makeover and watch how people begin to compliment you! You can begin your transformation by:

- Going shopping and trying on new clothes that you dreamed of wearing
- Developing a budget and finding reasonable items that mix-and-match
- Getting a haircut if you're a male
- Getting a pedicure, manicure, and facial
- Relaxing with an aromatherapy massage, accompanied by candles
- Treating yourself to a healthy snack or lunch at a place that has a great atmosphere
- Fasting and praying for a healthy, new you. Ask God to decrease your stress and give you the will power to change
- Inviting trustworthy people into your life, as you eliminate the negative people
- Writing down important goals and develop a plan to accomplish them
- Networking, especially if you're trying to connect in business
- Fellowshipping with family and friends
- Letting your hair down and laughing (it's God's cure for a broken heart.)
- Joining church and getting involved- complaining never changed anything

You deserve the very best! I started counting my blessings. Life is too short to stay depressed and angry. Let those family curses go and give your children to God! As parents you want the very best for your children, but sometimes they may get off track and cause you trauma and stress. In our relationships we want so desperately to change people, but the simple truth is that it is not our responsibility, only God can change them. Celebrate life and give birth to new beginnings, and lean towards a new life experience!

I'm sure you may ask what this information has to do with weight gain or being healthy. Well losing weight starts with the mind. Once you make your mind up, all else follows. Many people try to hold on to their impractical food cravings. I can recall telling myself every Monday that I was going to diet, but once that day came, I would mess up. Life kept getting in the way.

This list contains things that enable you to make excuses:

- I *have* to have my fried foods
- I need my coffee
- My caffeine helps me to get through the day
- Drinking relaxes me
- I'm on vacation; when I get back, I will cut back
- I am starving and I need to go grocery shopping
- My job keeps me so busy and I just grab anything
- I travel too much and the foods at the hotels aren't healthy
- I hate eating rabbit food
- Dieting is boring
- I have no idea what to eat
- Eating healthy foods are too expensive
- I don't eat that much so I have no idea why I'm not losing weight
- My family doesn't want to eat healthy

Have you ever made any of these excuses? If you have, make that necessary change today. You're worth it; let go of the complaining and being content. People would tell me how beautiful I was when I was over-weight, and it made me feel that it was okay to be over-weight. I was very unhealthy and borderline diabetic.

These are the changes I made:

- How I think
- I became focused on eating healthy
- I practiced self-control
- Learned how to be patient
- I became informed about healthy eating
- Focused on one thing at a time and gave it my all
- Stopped blaming others for my down falls
- Surrounded myself with people who celebrated me
- Became grateful for what I have, but continued to grow in business
- Thanked God for everything

Love yourself and take small steps into your new life. I used to set limits on what I could accomplish in life. After I lost the weight, I grew mentally. You can talk yourself out of a good thing or in to a good thing. I decided, along with God, how my future would be. If you want it, you can conquer it. If you are tired of things not working out for you, then change your universe. This may be an awakening for you; walk into your God given purpose today!

Everyday pray for God to order your steps, and watch positive things begin to happen for you. My life is beautiful. Now I look in the mirror and I love what I see inside and out! All of this transition took time. I fell off the wagon, but I got up, dusted myself off, and got back on track. Understand that falling is okay, but not getting up is a major problem. I now dress for success.

My mind has also lost weight. I lost negative thinking and that weighed tons! But I also gained weight in my mind. I gained the access to a powerful new world of information. The characters in the video "The Secret," gave testimonials and information about the universe that inspired me to surround myself with positive people and positive things. I learned a lot, but it was years before I put anything in to practice. My secret is King Jesus, and believing in myself. I remember listening to a video on forgiving people and the minister truly helped me. It wasn't until later that I understood what that meant. Now I refuse to let anyone pay free rent in my mind! I am fancy free spirit. I still go through things, but I knock down one problem at a time! I live, love, and stay healthy! I am truly LOVING the foods I use to hate, while living a diabetic, stress free life!

Glossary

Apple Cider Vinegar

Apple Cider Vinegar Cures

Apple Cider Vinegar, that wonderful old-timers home remedy, cures more ailments than any other folk remedy. It cures allergies (including pet, food and environmental), sinus infections, acne, high cholesterol, flu, chronic fatigue, candida, acid reflux, sore throats, contact dermatitis, arthritis, and gout. Apple Cider Vinegar also breaks down fat and is widely used to lose weight. It has also been reported that a daily dose of apple cider vinegar in water will have high blood pressure under control within two weeks [18].

Basil

Diabetes and Cardiovascular Disease

Basil extracts may also influence the development of two other major diseases currently affecting an enormous proportion of North Americans: diabetes and heart disease. Basil essential oils have been shown to lower blood glucose, triglyceride and cholesterol levels. Each of these has tremendous clinical implications.

Glucose, the main nutrient used by cells, is obtained from the digestive breakdown of food and is delivered to cells through the bloodstream. The pancreas secretes a crucial player involved in glucose delivery – insulin – to help regulate this movement of glucose into cells. Insulin's primary job is to transport glucose into cells so that it can be used or stored.

When blood glucose is high, the sugar can damage the body; in addition, the body keeps releasing insulin in an attempt to control blood sugar levels. Both high blood sugar and high insulin can do damage.

High blood glucose is a marker for diabetes, a chronic disease characterized by an impaired ability to produce or utilize insulin. Type 2 diabetes is more prevalent than type 1; type 2 diabetics can manage their condition through medication and, more importantly, through dietary and lifestyle modifications. With all of these lifestyle diseases, it's important to keep circulating glucose levels under control – both to prevent the harmful consequences of high blood sugar, as well as high levels of insulin as the body attempts to deal with blood glucose running amok.

This is where basil and other glucose-lowering agents come into play. Holy basil in particular has been found to reduce circulating glucose levels in both normal and diabetic laboratory animals as well as in diabetic humans. These results, particularly the evidence from human experiments, are hopeful and add credibility to the medicinal use of basil in ancient cultures. Although it is unclear which active compounds are responsible for basil's anti-diabetic effects, researchers think its essential oils are involved.

Basil's triglyceride- and cholesterol-lowering properties also offer promise for preventing cardiovascular disease. The combination of high circulating triglycerides (a form of fat in the blood) and LDL cholesterol (the "bad" kind that can clog blood vessels) are risk factors for atherosclerosis, heart attack and stroke. In an experiment in rats, sweet basil extracts hindered platelet aggregation (the clumping together of blood platelets to form a clot) and thrombosis (the actual formation of the blood clot), suggesting the potential for heart attack and stroke prevention. Although the research is still preliminary, basil shows therapeutic potential for cardiovascular disease prevention and treatment [17].

Nutrients in Basil
2.00 tsp. (2.80 grams)

Nutrient% Daily Value

Vitamin K 60%

Iron 6.5%

Calcium 5.9%

Vitamin A 5.2%

Fiber 4.5%

Manganese 4.5%

Tryptophan 3.1%

Vitamin B 63%

Magnesium 2.9%

Vitamin C 2.8%

This chart graphically details the %DV that a serving of Basil provides for each of the nutrients of which it is a good, very good, or excellent source according to our Food Rating System. Additional information about the amount of these nutrients provided by Basil can be found in the Food Rating System Chart. A link that takes you to the In-Depth Nutritional Profile for Basil, featuring information over 80 nutrients, can be found under the Food Rating System Chart [17].

Borage

Health Benefits of Borage

- Borage is one of very popular culinary herb especially in Mediterranean countries. The herb contains many notable phyto-nutrients, minerals, and vitamins that are essential for optimum health and wellness.
- The herb parts contain essential fatty acid gamma-linolenic acid (GLA), typically in concentrations of 17-20%. Linolenic acid is omega-6 fatty acid that play vital role in restoration of joint health, immunity, healthy skin and mucus membranes.
- Fresh *burrage* herb has high levels of vitamin C (ascorbic acid); provide 35 mcg or 60% of RDA per 100 g. Vitamin C is one of the powerful

natural anti-oxidant help remove harmful free radicals from the body. Along with other anti-oxidants, it has immune booster, wound healing and anti-viral effects.

- Burrage herb contains very high levels of vitamin A (140% of RDA) and carotenes. Both these compounds are powerful flavonoid anti-oxidants. Together, they act as protective scavengers against oxygen-derived free radicals and reactive oxygen species (ROS) that play a role in aging and various disease processes.
- Vitamin A is known to have antioxidant properties and is essential for vision. It is also required for maintaining healthy mucus membranes and skin. Consumption of natural foods rich in vitamin A and carotenes are known to help body protect from lung and oral cavity cancers.
- The herb has good amount of minerals like iron (41% of RDA), calcium, potassium, manganese, copper, zinc, and magnesium. Potassium is an important component of cell and body fluids, which helps control heart rate and blood pressure. Manganese is used by the body as a co-factor for the antioxidant enzyme, *superoxide dismutase.* Iron is an important co-factor for *cytochrome oxidase enzyme* in the cellular metabolism. In addition, being a component of hemoglobin inside the red blood cells, it determines the oxygen carrying capacity of the blood.
- The herb is one of the good sources of B-complex vitamins, particularly rich in niacin (vitamin B-3). Niacin helps lower LDL cholesterol levels in

the body. In addition, it has riboflavin, thiamin, pyridoxine, and folates in adequate levels. These vitamins function as co-factors in the enzymatic metabolism inside the body [3].

Burdock Root

Burdock Root Health Benefits

- Burdock roots, young shoots, peeled stalks, and dried seeds contain numerous compounds that are known to have anti-oxidant, disease preventing, and health promoting properties.
- The root is very low in calories; provides about 72 calories per 100 g. Burdock is very good source of many non-starch polysaccharides such as inulin, glucoside-lappin, mucilage...etc that help act as good laxative. In addition, inulin acts as prebiotic helps reduce blood sugar level, weight and cholesterol levels in the blood.
- Burdock root is especially containing good amounts of electrolyte potassium (308 mg or 6.5% of daily-required levels per 100 g root) and low in sodium. Potassium is an important component of cell and body fluids that helps control heart rate and blood pressure.
- It also contains some valuable minerals such as iron, manganese, magnesium; and small amounts of zinc, calcium, selenium, and phosphorus.
- This herb root contains small quantities of many vital vitamins including folic acid, riboflavin, pyridoxine, niacin, vitamin-E, and vitamin-C that are essential for optimum health. Both vitamin C and E is powerful natural antioxidants help body stave off infections, cancer and neurologic conditions [4].

Celery

Celery contains blood pressure reducing properties. It contains active compounds called Pthalides, which relax the muscles of the arteries that regulate blood pressure, allowing these vessels to dilate. Celery is also an excellent source of Vitamin C [20]

Chives

Chives belong to the onion family. They give a nice, zesty flavor to food. The plant is the smallest member of the family. It has long, narrow leaves attached to a slender bulb. You can use chives to flavor soups, stews, sauces and salads. It can also be used as a garnish. Chives are an excellent salt substitute and a perfect aid for those on a low fat, salt restricted diet. It contains vitamins A, B6, C and K. Several minerals are found in chives including calcium, copper, iron, magnesium, manganese, phosphorous, potassium, selenium and zinc. It is also a good source of folic acid and dietary fiber. The small, onion-like vegetable has several benefits to health [11].

Antibiotic

Like most plants in the allium group, chives have antibiotic properties. The natural antibacterial and antiviral agents in the vegetable work with vitamin C to destroy harmful microbes. This makes the plant an excellent natural defense against the common cold, flu and certain yeast infections.

Anti-Inflammatory

The plant has a mild anti-inflammatory effect. When included in your diet it can help reduce the risk of rheumatoid arthritis. The juice of the plant can be used as an insect repellent. When applied to wounds, it reduces fungal infections. The chive plant is rich in vitamin C which helps to prevent bruises and wounds. It also supports the immune system. Vitamin E in the plant has antioxidant properties which support the functions of the immune system. These vitamins also help to eradicate free radicals that can damage cells.

Anti-Carcinogenic

Chives are also used as a medicine. They help inhibit the growth of tumors and cancer. The small onions have been found helpful in the treatment of esophageal, stomach, prostrate and gastrointestinal tract cancers. Selenium in the small onion helps to protect cells from the effects of toxins and free radicals.

Circulatory

Flavonoids occur richly in this onion-like vegetable, helping to stabilize blood pressure and reduce hypertension. Sulfides in the plant help to lower blood lipids and blood pressure. Chives also contain substances that prevent blood clots. The high amounts of vitamin C in the plant help to improve the elasticity of blood capillaries. Folic acid helps to prevent constriction of blood vessels. This improves blood circulation. Vitamin C also facilitates absorption of iron in the body.

Cardiovascular

Regular intake of chives improves blood pressure. It also helps to reduce bad cholesterol levels. These beneficial effects on blood help to lower the risk of stroke and heart disease. The zesty vegetable helps to prevent calcification in arteries. Vitamin B6 reduces the levels of homcysteine in the blood. This is a product of cellular biochemical activity. High levels damage the walls of blood vessels. Selenium helps to prevent heart disease.

Digestion

Chives are an excellent source of dietary fiber. Plenty of roughage in the diet facilitates proper digestion. It contributes to intestinal health. This helps to prevent constipation and hemorrhoids. However, excessive consumption can unsettle the digestive system

Cilantro

Cilantro is a popular Mediterranean herb commonly recognized in Asia as coriander. It is widely employed in particularly savory dishes all cultures both in modern as well as traditional cuisines. The herb contains many notable plant derived chemical compounds that are known to have disease preventing and health-promoting properties. It is quite similar to dill in utility terms of its leaves and seeds which can be used as seasoning [5].

Ginger

Ginger can be used for a cold remedy to eliminate toxins and raise body heat. It may also be a blood thinner may reduce angina episodes by lowering cholesterol. The increase in blood flow helps relieve abdominal cramps and open the pelvis to bring on menstruation. Ginger also can help treat nausea, arthritis. It also speeds up the delivery of healthy plant chemicals into the blood stream [14].

Mint

Mint helps with digestive problems, and it may also relieve stomach aches. It has been known to relieve IBS (Irritable Bowel Syndrome), and reduce pain from headaches. Mint even helps migraines and infections in the body. Mint may help slow down bacteria and fungus growth in the body. It has been known to relax your mind and make you calm. Mint may also help prevent cancer [19].

Oregano

Oregano is known to have strong antibacterial properties, perhaps as a result of the volatile oils the herb contains. Some of these powerful volatile oils include thymol and carvacrol [10].

Parsley

Parsley is a bitter, aromatic, and diuretic herb that relaxes spasms, reduces inflammation and clears toxins. It is also said to inhibit tumor-cell growth and stimulates the digestion and uterus [15].

Peppermint

Peppermint can be used to soothe stomach ailments and other mild illnesses. It can also retard the growth of bacteria [1].

Rosemary herb

Properties and Benefits of Rosemary

Among the main properties of rosemary we can enumerate: analgesic, antiseptic, antidepressant, anti-inflammatory, expectorant, antiviral, aphrodisiac, disinfectant. Its active elements have choleric, antiseptic, diuretic and tonic aspects at a nervous level, stimulating bile secretion and eliminating it in the intestines, destroying microorganisms, increasing the quantity of eliminated urine, improving the blood flow and refreshing and energizing the mind. Apart from this, scientific researches indicate that rosemary is an ideal memory stimulant for both adults and students. Rosemary contains a series of secondary elements such as carnosol and carnosic acid, with a reflecting action in case of free radicals. Rosemary also has calming effects by working against fatigue, sadness, anxiety, calming muscle soreness, digestive pains and also, indigestion caused by stress [2].

Sage

Health Benefits

Like rosemary, its sister herb in the mint (*Labitae*) family, sage contains a variety of volatile oils, flavonoids (including *apigenin*, *diosmetin*, and *luteolin*), and phenolic acids, including the phenolic acid named after rosemary—*rosmarinic acid*.

Anti-Oxidant/Anti-Inflammatory Actions

Rosmarinic acid can be readily absorbed from the GI tract, and once inside the body, acts to reduce inflammatory responses by altering the concentrations of inflammatory messaging molecules (like leukotriene B4). The rosmarinic acid in sage and rosemary also functions as an antioxidant. The leaves and stems of the sage plant also contain antioxidant enzymes, including SOD (superoxide dismutase) and peroxidase. When combined, these three components of sage—flavonoids, phenolic acids, and oxygen-handling enzymes—give it a unique capacity for stabilizing oxygen-related metabolism and preventing oxygen-based damage to the cells. Increased intake of sage as a seasoning in food is recommended for persons with inflammatory conditions (like rheumatoid arthritis), as well as bronchial asthma, and atherosclerosis. The ability of sage to protect oils from oxidation has also led some companies to experiment with sage as a natural antioxidant additive to cooking oils that can extend shelf life and help avoid rancidity.

Better Brain Function

Want some sage advice? Boost your wisdom quotient by liberally adding sage to your favorite soups, stews and casserole recipes. Research published in the June 2003 issue of *Pharmacological Biochemical Behavior* confirms what herbalists have long known: sage is an outstanding memory enhancer. In this placebo-controlled, double-blind, crossover study, two trials were conducted using a total of 45 young adult volunteers. Participants were given either placebo or a standardized essential oil extract of sage in doses ranging from 50 to 150 microls. Cognitive tests were then conducted 1, 2, 4, 5, and 6 hours afterwards. In both trials, even the 50 microl dose of sage significantly improved subjects' immediate recall.

In other research presented at the British Pharmaceutical Conference in Harrogate (September 15-17, 2003), Professor Peter Houghton from King's College provided data showing that the dried root of *Salvia miltiorrhiza*, also known as Danshen or Chinese sage, contains active compounds similar to those developed into modern drugs used to treat Alzheimer's Disease. Sage has been used in the treatment of cerebrovascular disease for over one thousand years. Four compounds isolated from an extract from the root of Chinese sage were found to be acetylcholinesterase (AChE) inhibitors. The memory loss characteristic of Alzheimer's disease is accompanied by an increase of AChE activity that leads to its depletion from both cholinergic and noncholinergic neurons of the brain. Amyloid beta-protein (A beta), the major component of amyloid plaques which form in the brain in Alzeeimer's disease, acts on the expression of AChE, and AChE activity is increased around amyloid plaques. By inhibiting this increase in AChE activity, sage provides a useful therapeutic option to the use of pharmaceutical AChE inhibitors [6].

Spearmint

Health benefits of spearmint

- Spearmint is pleasantly aromatic herb packed with numerous health benefiting vitamins, antioxidants and phyto-nutrients.
- The leaves and herb parts contain essential oil menthol. However, unlike in peppermint, spearmint does not contain high amounts of menthol (0.5% compared to the 40% in peppermint), making it least pungent and subtly fragrant herb in mint family.
- The herb has low calories (about 43 cal per 100 g) and contains zero cholesterol.
- The chief essential oil in spearmint is menthol. Other important chemical components of spearmint are *α-pinene, β-pinene, carvone, cineole, linalool, limonene, myrcene* and *caryophyllene*. These compounds in mint help relieve fatigue and stress.
- The herb parts are also very good in minerals like potassium, calcium, manganese, iron, and magnesium. Iron is required for enzymes in cellular metabolism and synthesis of hemoglobin. Potassium in an important component of cell and body fluids that helps control heart rate and blood pressure. Manganese is used by the body as a co-factor for the antioxidant enzyme superoxide dismutase.
- It is also rich in many antioxidant vitamins including vitamin A (provides 4054 IU or 135% of RDA), beta carotene, vitamin C, folates (26% of RDA), vitamin B-6 (pyridoxine), riboflavin and thiamin.

Medicinal uses

Almost all parts of mint herb found place in various traditional as well in modern medicine.

- The herb decoction is an excellent remedy for minor ailments such as headaches, nervous strain, fatigue and stress, as well as for the respiratory problems; helping with asthma, bronchitis and catarrh.
- It is very useful to deal with digestive problems including nausea, flatulence and hiccups as it relaxes the stomach muscles.
- The essential oil, menthol, also has analgesic, local anaesthetic and counterirritant properties. Used in toothpaste and mouth refreshers.
- On the skin, when used as cream or lotion, it may help relieve the itching of pruritis, dermatitis and hives.
- Used as blended massage oil or in the aromatic therapy spearmint oil helps with headaches, stress, fatigue, and nervous conditions and to relieve itching.
- Spearmint tea can be used safely in pregnancy. In women, it helps reduce unwanted hairs through its anti-androgenic properties [7].

See the table below for in depth analysis of nutrients:

Spearmint (*Mentha spicata*), fresh,
Nutritional value per 100 g.
(Source: USDA National Nutrient data base)

Principle	Nutrient Value	Percentage of RDA
Energy	44 Kcal	2%
Carbohydrates	8.41 g	6.5%
Protein	3.29 g	6%
Total Fat	0.73 g	3%
Cholesterol	0 mg	0%
Dietary Fiber	6.8 g	18%
Vitamins		
Folates	105 mcg	26%
Niacin	0.948 mg	6%
Pyridoxine	0.158 mg	12%
Riboflavin	0.175 mg	13.5%
Thiamin	0.078 mg	6.5%
Vitamin A	4054 IU	135%
Vitamin C	13.3 mg	22%
Electrolytes		
Sodium	30 mg	2%
Potassium	458 mg	64%
Minerals		
Calcium	199 mg	20%
Copper	0.240 mg	75%
Iron	11.87 mg	148%
Magnesium	63 mg	16%
Manganese	1.118 mg	48.5%
Zinc	1.09 mg	10%

[7]

Stevia

Stevia is a plant that is grown in South America; it is commonly used as a sweetener. It is a natural way to add a healthy, natural sweetness to your food [8].

Sweet marjoram

It is an herb, which is one of the most sought after Mediterranean herbs known for its unique delicate flavor, fragrance, and anti- oxidant [9].

Tarragon

Tarragon is known as the King of herbs in France. Tarragon is rich in vitamins and phytonutrients that may impart health benefits, such as: tooth ache remedy and the decrease of sore gums. According to Sally Bernstein, a pain relieving effete, this is due to a substance called eugenol, which is found in clove oil [13].

Thyme herb

Health Benefits of Thyme Herb

- Thyme contains many active principles that are found to have disease preventing and health promoting properties.
- Thyme herb contains thymol, one of the important essential oils, which scientifically have been found to have antiseptic, anti-fungal characteristics. The other volatile oils in thyme include *carvacolo, borneol* and *geraniol*.

- Thyme contains many flavonoid Phenolic antioxidants like *zeaxanthin, lutein, pigenin, naringenin, luteolin,* and *thymonin.* Fresh thyme herb has one of the highest antioxidant levels among herbs, a total ORAC (Oxygen Radical Absorbance Capacity) value of 27426-umol TE/100 g.
- Thyme is packed with minerals and vitamins that are essential for optimum health. Its leaves are one of the richest sources of potassium, iron, calcium, manganese, magnesium, and selenium. Potassium is an important component of cell and body fluids that helps controlling heart rate and blood pressure. Manganese is used by the body as a co-factor for the antioxidant enzyme, *superoxide dismutase.* Iron is required for red blood cell formation.
- The herb is also a rich source of many important vitamins such as B-complex vitamins, beta carotene, vitamin A, vitamin K, vitamin E, vitamin C and folic acid.
- Thyme provides 0.35 mg of vitamin B-6 or pyridoxine; furnishing about 27% of daily recommended intake. Pyridoxine keeps up GABA (beneficial neurotransmitter in the brain) levels in the brain, which has stress buster function.
- Vitamin C helps body develop resistance against infectious agents and scavenge harmful, pro-inflammatory free radicals.
- Vitamin A is a fat soluble vitamin and antioxidant that is required maintaining healthy mucus membranes and skin and is also essential for vision. Consumption of natural foods rich in flavonoids like vitamin A and beta-carotene helps protect from lung and oral cavity cancers.

Thyme leaves offer significant levels of quality phyto-nutrients profile. Just 100g of fresh leaves provides (% of Recommended daily allowance)

38% of dietary fiber
27% of vitamin B-6 (pyridoxine)
266% of vitamin C
158% of vitamin A
218% of iron
40% of calcium
40% of magnesium
75% of manganese
but no cholesterol [12].

See the table below for in depth analysis of nutrients:

Thyme herb (Thymus vulgaris), Fresh leaves,
Nutritive value per 100 g. ORAC value 27426,
(Source: USDA National Nutrient data base)

Principle	Nutrient Value	Percentage of RDA
Energy	101 Kcal	5%
Carbohydrates	24.45 g	18%
Protein	5.56 g	10%
Total Fat	1.68 g	8.4%
Cholesterol	0 mg	0%
Dietary Fiber	14.0 g	37%
Vitamins		
Folates	45 mcg	11%
Niacin	1.824 mg	11%
Pantothenic acid	0.409 mg	8%
Pyridoxine	0.348 mg	27%
Riboflavin	0.471 mg	36%
Thiamin	0.48 mg	4%
Vitamin A	4751 IU	158%
Vitamin C	160.1 mg	266%
Electrolytes		
Sodium	9 mg	0.5%
Potassium	609 mg	13%
Minerals		
Calcium	405 mg	40.5%
Iron	17.45 mg	218%
Magnesium	160 mg.	40%
Manganese	1.719 mg	75%
Manganese	106 mg	15%

Zinc	1.81 mg	16.5%
Phyto-nutrients		
Carotene-ß	2851 mcg	--

[12]

Turmeric

It is a bitter herb that has a pungent smell, with astringent, anti-biotic, anti-inflammatory and anticoagulant properties. It is used to stimulate the uterus, digestive, respiratory and circulate systems. Turmeric normalizes dry energy flow and lowers cholesterol levels.

The herb helps with digestive problems and skin complaints, circulatory disorders, as well as tumors in the uterus and menstrual problems [16].

Cooking with herbs is more than a good thing; it is God's gift to you. Not only do herbs play a healing role in your body, but they taste good as well. Many people tend to take the easy way by not reading labels, or even knowing the consequences of a poor diet.

Join my team of boot campers who love my mouthwatering foods!!!

For more information, log on to:

www.livingdiabeticfree.com

Special Thanks

I want to thank God for ordering my steps and blessing this opportunity!

I want to thank my husband, Mr. Perry C. Brown, for his love and support. Thank you Perry for giving my book cover a professional, but artistic, elegant flare! I will never forget your passion for my dreams! THANK YOU SOUL MATE! I love you Poppy!

I want to thank my step-son, Perry Brown for being a blessing in my life and a good son. I love you handsome!

I want to thank my cousin Tameka Key Woods, you gave me a wonderful gift; I will never forget it!

I want to thank Marisa Johnson. Thank you for encouraging me to stay focused and write my book. I will always be grateful for your faith in me! May God bless you and give you favor for life! You are a diva with a beautiful heart!

I want to thank Mr. and Mrs. Hancock. You both saw my vision and you gave it your all!

I want to thank all my family and friends who supported me!

I want to thank Shanel Johnson, my editor. You have embraced my book and I am very pleased. I want a very long business relationship. I know God put us together and He never makes mistakes! Your career as an editor is very long and promising. I pray you stay a beautiful Angel! You took the time to make it a success! I celebrate this moment with you!

Contact

Angela H. Brown

cherrywinepublisher@yahoo.com

www.livingdiabeticfree.com for booking information

901-314-9806

Deana Taylor

finallyfitmem@yahoo.com

www.finallyfitmemphis.com

www.facebook.com/deanadtaylor

www.twitter.com/deanadtaylor

Dr. Howard Nelson

www.comprehensiveprofessionalservices.net

Office (901-729-1900)

Mobile (901-596-6234)

kac0020@hotmail.com

Hancock Photography and Videographer

(901) 345-0334

Artistic Impressions Photography- Perry Brown

perry_brownsr@yhaoo.com

www.linkedin.com/perrycbrown

www.facebook.com/artisticimpressionsphotagraphy

901-314-9828

Professhanel Editing - Shanel Johnson

ShanelDJ@hotmail.com

(901) 687-7185

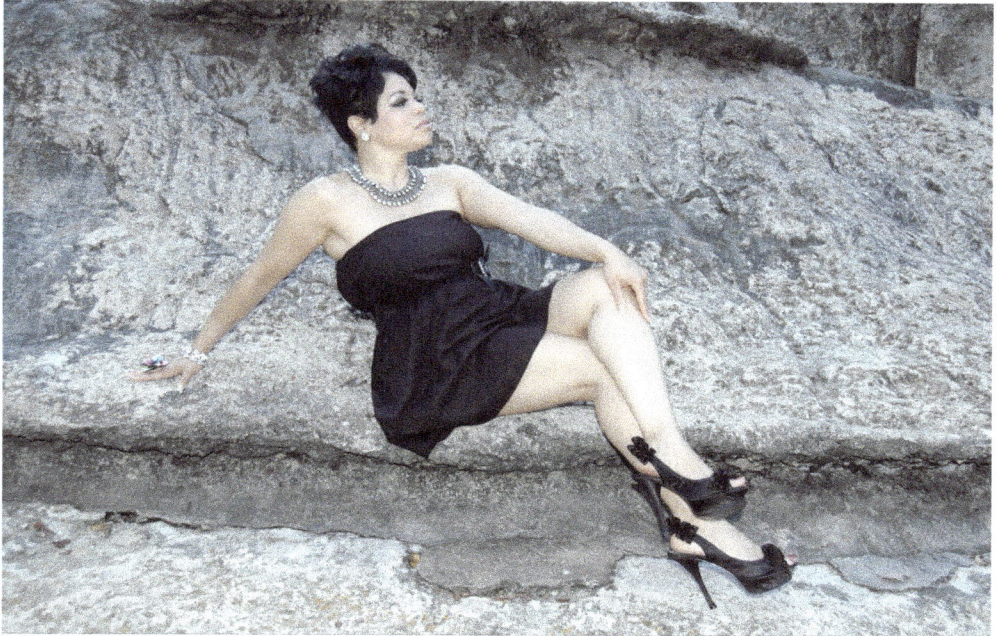

Angela H. Brown is now celebrating an exciting makeover - inside and out. Her secret for a beautiful look is, Arbornne! Angela enjoys a chemical-sulfate free makeup line, which enhances her natural beauty, while leaving her skin feeling like silk! If you want to experience this new lifestyle, then indulge without the guilt. Ladies: take a tour and check out the beauty products that will make you feel brand new, and explore some of the healthy items for the kids as well. Men: shaving will now leave you feeling suave and smooth, and if you're working out, check out the quick, delicious fat burning shakes.

Log onto www.arbornne.com

My user ID# is 13144674

Notes

1. Anonymous. "Benefits of Peppermint" Health By Nature. August 17, 2012. http://nature2health.blogspot.com/2012/08/benefits-of-peppermint.html
2. Anonymous. "Benefits of Rosemary Herb" Live and Feel. 2006. http://www.liveandfeel.com/medicinalplants/rosemary.html
3. Anonymous. "Borage Nutrition Facts" Power Your Diet. 2009. http://www.nutrition-and-you.com/borage.html
4. Anonymous. "Burdock Root Nutrition Facts" Power Your Diet. 2009. http://www.nutrition-and-you.com/burdock-root.html
5. Anonymous. "Cilantro (Coriander) Nutrition Facts" Power Your Diet. 2000. http://www.nutrition-and-you.com/cilantro.html
6. Anonymous. "Health Benefits" The World's Healthiest Foods. 2001. http://www.whfoods.com/genpage.php?pfriendly=1&tname=foodspice&dbid=76
7. Anonymous. "Spearmint Nutrition Facts" Power Your Diet. 2009. http://www.nutrition-and-you.com/spearmint.html
8. Anonymous. "Stevia Plant (herb) Nutrition Facts" Power Your Diet. 2009. http://www.nutrition-and-you.com/stevia-plant.html
9. Anonymous. "Sweet Marjoram Nutrition Facts" Power Your Diet. 2009. http://www.nutrition-and-you.com/sweet-marjoram.html
10. Anonymous. "The Benefits of Oregano" A 2 Z of Health, Beaut and Fitness. October 19, 2012. http://health.learninginfo.org/oregano.htm
11. Anonymous. "The Nutrition of Chives" FitDay. 2000. http://www.fitday.com/fitness-articles/nutrition/healthy-eating/the-nutrition-of-chives.html
12. Anonymous. "Thyme Herb Nutrition Facts" Power Your Diet. 2009. http://www.nutrition-and-you.com/thyme-herb.html

13. Banar, Maura. "What Are The Health Benefits of Tarragon?" LiveStrong. July 24, 2011. http://www.livestrong.com/article//
14. Julian, Marei. "Ginger Root & Its Many Health Benefits" Examiner. May 9, 2012. http://www.examiner.com/article/ginger-root-its-many-health-benefits
15. Meyer, Michael. "Parsley (rock selinon) Petroselinum Crispum" Ageless. January 8, 2012. http://www.ageless.co.za/herb-parsley.htm
16. Meyer, Michael. "Turmeric (Yu Jin) Curcuma longa (C. domestica)" Ageless. January 8, 2012. http://www.ageless.co.za/herb-turmeric.htm
17. O'brien, Paul. "What's So Healthy About Basil?" Precision Nutrition. November 11, 2009. http://www.precisionnutrition.com/healthy-basil
18. Power, Ikan. "Apple Cider Vinegar Cures." Little Drops of Water. January 26, 2012. http://www.ikanpower.com/apple-cidar-venigar-cures/
19. Vann, Madeline. "4 Natural Remedies for Nausea" Everyday Health. January 17, 2012. http://www.everydayhealth.com/digestive-health/four-natural-remedies-for-nausea.aspx
20. Wilson, Pat. "Think Celery" WeightLossResources. 2000. http://www.weightlossresources.co.uk/diet/healthy_eating/celery.htm

www.ingramcontent.com/pod-product-compliance
Lightning Source LLC
Chambersburg PA
CBHW070929270326
41927CB00011B/2782